RECOGNITION OF *M. LEPRAE* ANTIGENS

DEVELOPMENTS IN HEMATOLOGY AND IMMUNOLOGY

Lijnen, H.R., Collen, D. and Verstraete, M., eds: Synthetic Substrates in Clinical Blood Coagulation Assays. 1980. ISBN 90-247-2409-0

Smit Sibinga, C.Th., Das, P.C. and Forfar, J.O., eds: Paediatrics and Blood Transfusion. 1982. ISBN 90-247-2619-0

Fabris, N., ed: Immunology and Ageing. 1982. ISBN 90-247-2640-9

Hornstra, G.: Dietary Fats, Prostanoids and Arterial Thrombosis. 1982. ISBN 90-247-2667-0

Smit Sibinga, C.Th., Das, P.C. and Loghem, van J.J., eds: Blood Transfusion and Problems of Bleeding. 1982. ISBN 90-247-3058-9

Dormandy, J., ed: Red Cell Deformability and Filterability. 1983. ISBN 0-89838-578-4

Smit Sibinga, C.Th., Das, P.C. and Taswell, H.F., eds: Quality Assurance in Blood Banking and Its Clinical Impact. 1984. ISBN 0-89838-618-7

Besselaar, A.M.H.P. van den, Gralnick, H.R. and Lewis, S.M., eds: Thromboplastin Calibration and Oral Anticoagulant Control. 1984. ISBN 0-89838-637-3

Fondu, P. and Thijs, O., eds: Haemostatic Failure in Liver Disease. 1984. ISBN 0-89838-640-3

Smit Sibinga, C.Th., Das, P.C. and Opelz, G., eds: Transplantation and Blood Transfusion. 1984. ISBN 0-89838-686-1

Schmid-Schönbein, H., Wurzinger, L.J. and Zimmerman, R.E., eds: Enzyme Activation in Blood-Perfused Artificial Organs. 1985. ISBN 0-89838-704-3

Dormandy, J., ed: Blood Filtration and Blood Cell Deformability. 1985. ISBN 0-89838-714-0

Smit Sibinga, C.Th., Das, P.C. and Seidl, S., eds: Plasma Fractionation and Blood Transfusion. 1985. ISBN 0-89838-761-2

Dawids, S. and Bantjes, A., eds: Blood Compatible Materials and their Testing. 1986. ISBN 0-89838-813-9

Smit Sibinga, C.Th., Das, P.C. and Greenwalt, T.J., eds: Future Developments in Blood Banking. 1986. ISBN 0-89838-824-4

Berlin, A., Dean, J., Draper, M.H., Smith, E.M.B. and Spreafico, F., eds: Immunotoxicology. 1987. ISBN 0-89838-843-0

Ottenhoff, T. and De Vries, R.: Recognition of *M. leprae* antigens. 1987. ISBN 0-89838-887-2

Recognition of *M. leprae* antigens

by

TOM OTTENHOFF M.D.

Department of Immunohematology and Blood Bank, University Hospital,
Leiden, The Netherlands and
Armauer Hansen Research Institute,
Addis Abeba, Ethiopia

RENÉ DE VRIES M.D.

Department of Immunohematology and Blood Bank,
University Hospital, Leiden,
The Netherlands

1987 **MARTINUS NIJHOFF PUBLISHERS**
a member of the KLUWER ACADEMIC PUBLISHERS GROUP
DORDRECHT / BOSTON / LANCASTER

Distributors

for the United States and Canada: Kluwer Academic Publishers, P.O. Box 358, Accord Station, Hingham, MA 02018-0358, USA
for the UK and Ireland: Kluwer Academic Publishers, MTP Press Limited, Falcon House, Queen Square, Lancaster LA1 1RN, UK
for all other countries: Kluwer Academic Publishers Group, Distribution Center, P.O. Box 322, 3300 AH Dordrecht, The Netherlands

Library of Congress Cataloging in Publication Data

```
Ottenhoff, Tom.
   Recognition of M. leprae antigens.

   (Developments in hematology and immunology)
   1. Leprosy--Immunological aspects.  2. Leprosy--
Genetic aspects.  3. Leprosy--Diagnosis.  4. Bacterial
antigens.  I. Vries, René R. P. de.  II. Title.
III. Series.  [DNLM: 1. Antigens, Bacterial--immunology.
2. Mycobacterium Leprae--immunology.  W1 DE997VZK /
QW 125.5.M9 O89r]
RC154.O88   1987            616.9'9807          87-7753
```


ISBN-13: 978-94-010-7994-5   e-ISBN-13: 978-94-009-3327-9
DOI: 10.1007/978-94-009-3327-9

Copyright

CONTENTS

ABBREVIATIONS

AA	auto-immune arthritis
APC	antigen presenting cell
BB	(mid) borderline leprosy
BL	borderline lepromatous leprosy
BT	borderline tuberculoid leprosy
CMI	cell mediated immunereactivity
cpm	counts per minute
DTH	delayed type hypersensitivity
EBV-BC	Epstein-Barr virus transformed B cell line
H-2	histocompatibility system-2; the murine MHC
HS	human serum
HLA	human leucocyte antigen; the human MHC
γ IFN	gamma interferon
IL-2	interleukin-2
IMDM	Iscove's modified Dulbecco's medium
Ir gene	immune response gene
Is gene	immune suppression gene
K	kilodalton
LL	lepromatous leprosy
LTT	lymphocyte transformation test
MHC	major histocompatibility complex
M. leprae	*Mycobacterium leprae*
moab	monoclonal antibody
M_r	relative molecular mass
PBMNC	peripheral blood mononuclear cells
PHA	phytohaemagglutinin
PPD	purified protein derivative of *M. tuberculosis*
RA	rheumatoid arthritis
RD	restriction determinant
reglr gene	immune regulator gene
%RSAG	percentage relative antigenic stimulation
RR	relative risk
Tc	cytotoxic T lymphocyte
Th	helper T lymphocyte
Ts	suppressor T lymphocyte
TCL	T (lymphocyte) cell line
TLC	T lymphocyte clone
TT	tuberculoid leprosy

FOREWORD

Those who have had the privilege to visit the Sistine Chapel may remember the fresco painting of Jesus curing the leper (Marcus 1, 40-45). It seems that leprosy was not only known 2000 years ago but was also recognized as an important problem. Unfortunately, little has changed since then.

Although leprosy is mainly known as an "import" disease in Europe and North America, in the greater part of the world it remains the problem it has always been, one of a stigmatizing disease comparable to the modern day pestilence, namely AIDS. Who could forget Dürer's etch of a leper walking with a clapper to announce his presence, or the heartbreaking stories of patients, especially those with lepromatous leprosy, ousted by their own families to become social outcasts forced to beg for their food. This attitude is slowly changing and with this change the name of Mahatma Ghandi will always be connected and remembered.

There have been important breakthroughs in understanding the cause of the disease and its pathogenesis. Armauer Hansen's brilliant, clear and convincing description of what is known as *Mycobacterium leprae* heralded the beginning of a new era in the fight against leprosy. Once the cause was known, leprosy became less frightening, at least to the medical world. The hope that the battle against leprosy could be won was further strengthened when it was shown that simple hygiene could prevent the spread of the disease. This was further confirmed when autochthonous leprosy dissappeared from Europe altogether whereby improvement of the socio-economic situation certainly played an important role.

In most parts of the world the prospects remained grim until the nineteen-thirties when the introduction of DDS opened up the possibility to really "cure" the disease. The WHO launched a worldwide campaign against leprosy and over 100 million US dollars where spent trying to eradicate the disease. However, even with the arrival of newer and more powerful anti-mycobacterial drugs such as streptomycin, the disease remained steadfast. This was mainly due to two factors. The first being that the hygienic and socio-economic situation had not improved sufficiently, and secondly that no effective vaccine could be developed.

The underlying reason for this was an incomplete knowledge of the pathogenesis of the disease, and the immunological and genetic mechanisms which influence its course. *Mycobacterium leprae* can be seen as an intelligent parasite in the sense that the mycobacterium uses the immunological and other defence mechanisms of the host for its own ends without killing the host too quickly. Only when we fully understand how the mycobacterium does this will we be able to conquer leprosy.

This book describes a turning point in the continuing battle. It brings together the latest information from all over the world on the immunology and genetics of leprosy and contains important original work by two authors who may be considered to belong to the pioneers in this field. It provides important new insights, the relevance of which extends well beyond leprosy. The use of T cell (lymphocyte) clones has enabled the pathogenesis of leprosy to be unravelled to a large extent and has opened the way not only for a complete description of the different stages of the disease but also to development of effective and safe vaccines. The approach followed by the authors may, however, also be applied to other infectious diseases such as tuberculosis and AIDS, as well as auto-immune diseases like rheumatoid arthritis, type I diabetes and multiple sclerosis in which T cells also play a central role.

J.J. VAN ROOD

CHAPTER 1

INTRODUCTION

I. The immune system

The primary task of the immune system is the induction and regulation of protective immune responses against antigens that can threaten the individuals' self-integrity by causing disease (e.g. bacteria, viruses and other micro-organisms). In principle, all molecules and structures are antigenic and thus are capable of inducing immune responses. In order to maintain this self-integrity however, a second and essential prerequisite has to be fulfilled, namely the development and maintenance of tolerance against those antigenic structures of which the individuals' own body is composed. Immune responses against such self- or auto-antigens would result in undesired tissue damage and thus auto-immune disease.

The immune system consists of a complex network of closely cooperating cells and molecules, organized in distinct but related compartments distributed all over the body. One component of the immune system is predominantly antigen non-specific in its function. This component consists of phagocytic cells such as neutrophilic granulocytes, macrophages and monocytes which can phagocytize and subsequently kill micro-organisms, for instance bacteria; natural killer cells which presumably are involved in the killing of virally infected cells and malignantly transformed targets; and killer cells which are capable of directly lysing antibody coated target cells; in addition several soluble factors are involved like the complement products which can induce chemotaxis of cells as well as opsonization and lysis of e.g. bacteria and the several acute phase proteins produced during infection. Usually, the natural biochemical and physical barriers of ecto- and entodermal origin are not reckoned among the immune system, although they constitute an important line of primary defence against penetrating external antigens.

The other component of the immune system is essentially antigen specific in its function. To this end, the immune system has at its disposal a large repertoire of antigen specific receptors. One such a receptor in principle is able to recognize only one antigenic determinant. Once a first encounter with a particular antigen has taken place and has been followed by an adequate primary immune response, this antigen specific response is imprinted in the memory of the immune system. Upon second and subsequent antigen exposures, a secondary immune response evolves with greater efficiency and rapidity than the primary one. Secondary responses and immunological memory are characteristic only for the antigen specific immune system.

Antigen specific responses can be either humoral or cellular or both. The humoral immune response is mediated via B lymphocytes that express – clonally distributed – antigen receptors on their cell surface, namely immunoglobulins.

Following stimulation with the appropriate antigen, a B lymphocyte will proliferate and differentiate into a plasma cell secreting immunoglobulin with that particular specificity. The cellular immune response is mediated by T lymphocytes. At least three distinct T lymphocyte populations have been recognized, namely cytotoxic (Tc), helper (Th) and suppressor (Ts) T lymphocytes. Tc, Th and probably Ts express clonotypic (i.e. confined to the progeny of one single cell only) antigen receptors. In contrast however to the B lymphocyte antigen receptor which is a membrane bound immunoglobulin, Tc and Th antigen receptors cannot be activated by antigen alone. The antigen has to be presented to the T cell in association with a self-major histocompatibility complex (MHC) molecule on the membrane of an antigen presenting cell (ACP). The two groups of MHC molecules involved in antigen presentation, designated class I and class II molecules, are composed of both constant and variable or polymorphic domains, the latter of which are involved in the MHC restriction of antigen specific T cell activation.

Tc usually are activated by antigen in association with a self MHC class I molecule i.e. Tc are MHC class I restricted. Upon activation, Tc precursor cells proliferate and differentiate into effector Tc which are able to lyse target cells bearing the appropriate antigen – MHC class I complex. Such target cells include virally infected cells, hapten-modified target cells, cells carrying non-self transplantation antigens and tumor cells.

In contrast to Tc, Th recognize antigen in the context of a self MHC class II molecule. Activated Th cells can mediate both delayed type hypersensitivity (DTH) reactions and protective immunity against intracellular micro-organisms such as mycobacteria. In addition, Th lymphocytes initiate and regulate immune responses and consequently have a central position in the immune network. These regulatory Th functions include the amplification of antigen specific proliferation and differentiation of pre-Tc into Tc effector cells, the amplification of antigen driven expansion and maturation of B cells into plasma cells, the regulation of effector Th cells conferring DTH and protective immunity, and – probably – the induction of Ts cells. This latter group of T cells has been poorly characterized so far with respect to antigen receptors, MHC restriction and function, and even has remained the subject of debate regarding its existence. It is assumed that Ts cells represent a counterpart for Th cells in that they actively downregulate immune responses. Ts functions probably further include the maintenance of self-tolerance as well as the protection against diseases which can be the result of ongoing immune responses. The Ts cells have been subdivided in distinct subpopulations and may be more heterogeneous in nature than Th or Tc cells.

Thus, Th cells have a key role in the generation and amplification of antigen specific immune responses. The relevance of MHC class II restricted antigen specific Th cell activation probably correlates with the selective expression of class II molecules on immunocompetent, i.c. antigen presenting cells. Since Th cells will thus be unable to respond to freely circulating antigens as well as antigens on class II negative cells (these latter antigens may include auto-antigens which therefore remain hidden for Th cells), and can only be activated by antigen on the surface of specialized class II positive APC, Th cell activation may be limited and focussed only to relevant immunological areas. This constraint on Th cell activation may be important with regard to tolerance to auto-antigens as well as protection against tissue damage caused by uncontrolled Th cell reactivity. In contrast, MHC class I molecules are expressed on virtually all nucleated cells. MHC class I restricted Tc cells in principle therefore are able to recognize antigen on any relevant, e.g. virally infected, target cell when properly helped by Th cells, and thus can effectively attack target cells at any site of the body.

II. Antigen specific MHC immune response (Ir) genes

The ability of an individual to generate immune responses is controlled by a large number of different genes. Most of these genes are not related to the MHC, and are antigen non-specific, that is: they control immune responsiveness against a wide variety of unrelated antigens. For example, in mice a gene located on chromosome 1 determines the natural resistance or susceptibility to a number of unrelated intracellular micro-organisms.

Antigen specific immune response (Ir) genes were discovered when experimental animals were immunized with antigens carrying a highly restricted number of immunogenic determinants. Detailed analyses mapped these genes to the MHC. These genes therefore were designated MHC Ir genes. These Ir genes subsequently were shown to control only the response to so-called T cell dependent antigens. A series of elegant studies established that the products of the MHC Ir genes are the highly polymorphic MHC class I and class II molecules, and that these molecules control T cell dependent immune responses actually by restricting and regulating antigen specific T cell responsiveness.

Thus, the MHC class I and class II molecules are not only strong histocompatibility antigens in allogeneic tissue transplantation but also function as restriction and regulation elements for antigen specific T cells. Moreover, the extensive polymorphism of the MHC class I and II genes may directly explain the observed interindividual differences in antigen specific immune responsiveness. These interindividual differences in immune responsiveness controlled by HLA class I or II genes may result in differential susceptibility to or expression of disease. Many of the observed associations between HLA (the human MHC) alleles and several – mostly auto-immune – diseases are thought to reflect such HLA class I or II Ir gene controlled antigen specific differences in immune responsiveness. Thus, in resemblance to the situation in animal models, it is supposed that HLA class I or II (Ir) genes may control disease susceptibility by regulating immune responsiveness to the causative antigens. However, the fact that the supposed triggering antigens for the HLA associated diseases have remained unknown in many cases such as in auto-immune diseases, has hampered further studies on the nature of HLA Ir genes and the way in which they control immune responsiveness in relation to disease.

III. HLA class II and leprosy

Leprosy is a chronic infectious disease caused by *Mycobacterium leprae*. Acquired specific immunity against the bacillus closely correlates with Th cell mediated immunity. Th cell mediated immunity is present in the tuberculoid (TT) pole or type of the disease, but absent in the lepromatous (LL) one, presumably as a consequence of Ts mediated antigen specific suppression. HLA class II alleles are associated with leprosy type as well as with differential DTH reactivity against *M. leprae*, suggesting that these polymorphic class II alleles may be markers for HLA-linked *M. leprae* Ir genes. Since in the case of this HLA-disease association a) the triggering foreign antigen is known and b) the responsible antigen specific immune cells, namely Th, can be isolated, leprosy has been used as a human model in order to establish whether HLA class II molecules can be defined as the products of HLA class II linked Ir genes for *M. leprae*.

IV. Aims and outline of the studies

The aims of the studies presented here have been:
I. to define the antigenic determinants expressed by *M. leprae* that are recognized by Th and Ts cells from leprosy patients in order to characterize the T cell activating antigens which may be under HLA class II Ir/Is gene control;
II. to define the determinants on HLA class II molecules that restrict the *M. leprae* induced activation of Th cells from leprosy patients and healthy individuals.
III. to investigate whether HLA class II allele specific differences in the restriction of *M. leprae* reactive Th cell activation can be detected in a population where that particular allele is associated with TT leprosy; such a preferential restriction may be helpful in elucidating the mechanism(s) of HLA class II Ir gene effects.

After this introduction, an overview of the MHC class II genes and molecules, MHC class II restricted and Ir gene controlled T cell activation and leprosy as a model for the study of HLA class II Ir and Is genes in human diseases is given in chapter 2. In the following 2 chapters, several *M. leprae* antigenic determinants which can activate Th as well as Ts cells are described. In chapter 5, the HLA class II restriction determinants for *M. leprae* reactive Th cells from leprosy patients are characterized. Chapter 6 describes studies that concentrated on HLA-DR3 molecules as the products of a *M. leprae* class II (regulatory)

Ir gene predisposing to TT leprosy. The following chapter reports the results from skin test studies in LL and TT patients and discusses their relevance with regard to a second disease where HLA class II Ir genes may be important, namely rheumatoid arthritis. In the general discussion (chapter 8) the major findings of these studies are summarized and discussed with respect to their significance for leprosy and other HLA class II associated diseases.

CHAPTER 2

MHC CLASS II Ir/Is GENE CONTROLLED ANTIGEN SPECIFIC T CELL ACTIVATION AND DISEASE SUSCEPTIBILITY: LEPROSY, A HUMAN MODEL.

This chapter reviews several major aspects of the genetic control of the immune response by MHC class II Ir and Is genes followed by an overview of the immunology of leprosy with special emphasis on the role of HLA linked Ir and Is genes. The molecular and genomic organization of the MHC and the restriction of helper T cell activation by MHC class II molecules are the two topics to be discussed first. The third part summarizes in brief some hallmarks of the work on MHC class II Ir and Is genes in experimental animals, followed by a more detailed account of the evidence for human MHC class II Ir and Is genes. The final section of this chapter describes the different clinical manifestations of leprosy, the major immuneregulatory disturbances in the disease and the role of HLA linked (Ir and Is) genes in controlling the type of immune responsiveness and thus the type of leprosy that is mounted by the host against *Mycobacterium leprae*.

I. Genes and products of the major histocompatibility complex (MHC) in mouse and man

In the 1950's it became clear that multiple blood transfusions and pregnancies could induce the formation of antibodies against alloantigens expressed by leucocytes (1-4). Systematic analyses revealed that these human leucocyte antigens behaved as the products of allelic genes (5,6) situated at closely linked loci (7,8), and that they were strong histocompatibility antigens in allogeneic tissue transplantation (9,10). The tight linkage of these loci led to the notion of a single complex genetic system, which appeared to be strikingly homologous between different mammalian species (11) and was designated major histocompatibility complex (MHC). The human and the murine MHC, respectively called HLA and H-2, have been studied in the most detail by means of various serological, cellular and finally biochemical techniques. These studies have led to the identification of a large number of MHC genes and products (figure 1).

The HLA genomic region is located on the short arm of the 6th chromosome and encodes two major types of products, the class I and class II molecules (12,13). These two groups of molecules show homologies as well as differences in structure and function (13). Besides the class I and class II genes, a number of other genes has been mapped into the HLA region, namely several complement

13

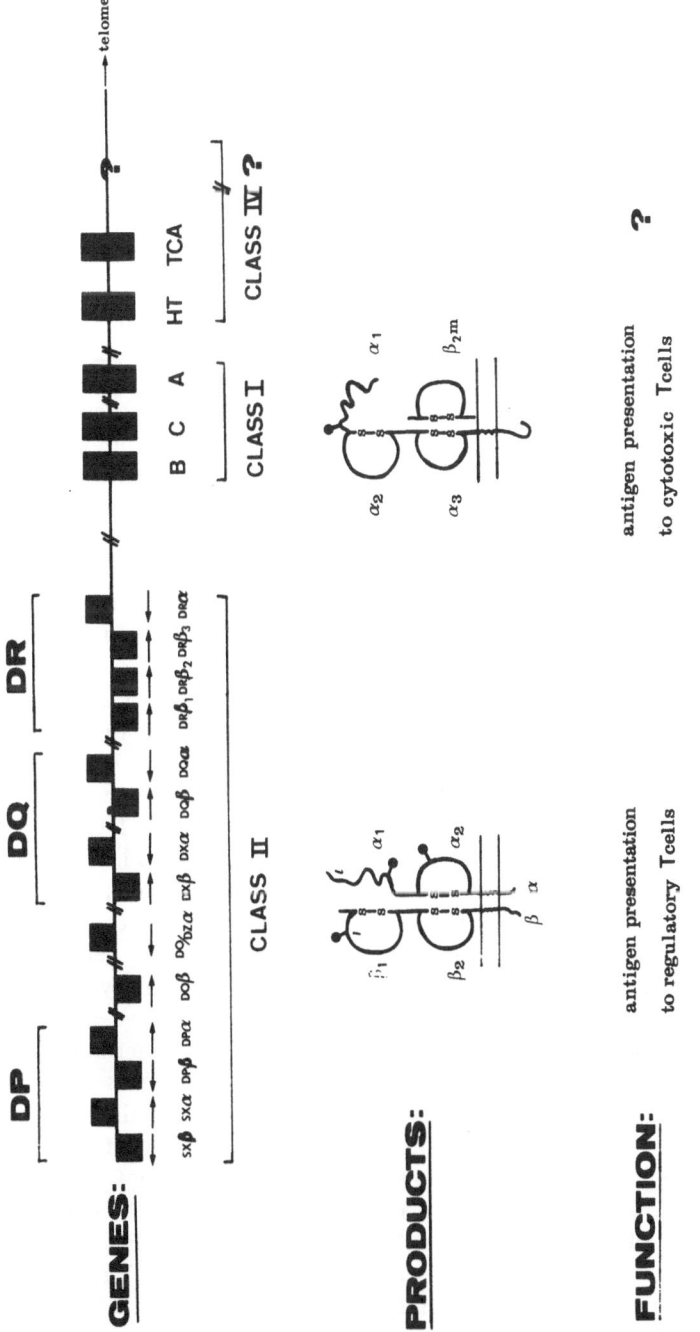

Fig. 1
Schematic representation of the genomic organization of the HLA region on chromosome 6.

(C2, Bf, C4A, C4B) or class III genes coding for complement factors (14) and two 21 steroidhydroxylase (21OH-A, 21OH-B) genes (15). The relationship of these genes and their products to the class I and class II ones has remained unclear, and will not be discussed here. (For a review, the reader may be referred to ref. 14).

HLA class I molecules are highly polymorphic membrane glycoproteins coded by three distinct multi-allelic loci namely HLA-A, -B and -C. These molecules are composed of a heavy and a light chain which are non-covalently linked. The heavy or α chain (M_r: 44K) is folded into 3 extra-cellular domains designated α_1, α_2 and α_3 and possesses a transmembrane region and a cytoplasmic tail in addition (reviewed in 16). The membrane proximal α_3 domain is non-covalently associated with the light chain, called β_2 microglobulin. β_2m (M_r: 12K) is encoded by a gene on chromosome 15 (17), and is composed of a single domain, but does not penetrate the cell membrane. Class I molecules are expressed by nearly all nucleated cells. The extensive allelic polymorphism is expressed by the α_1 and α_2 domains (18). The α_3 domain shows sequence homology with β_2m as well as with the constant domains of other membrane proteins belonging to the so called immunoglobulin superfamily such as class II molecules, T cell receptor chains, immunoglobulins, CD8 molecules and several other membrane molecules (19).

HLA class II molecules are expressed as heterodimeric glycoproteins consisting of a heavy (α; M_r: 33-35K) and a light (β; M_r 26-29K) chain, joined on the cell surface by non-covalent bonds. Each chain consists of 2 extracellular domains (respectively α_1, α_2, β_1 and β_2) which in part are held together by disulfide bridges, as is the case for class I domains. Both class II chains penetrate the cell membrane and possess an intracytoplasmic part (reviewed in 20-22). The genomic class II organization is more complex than that of the HLA-A, -B, -C region. At least four gene clusters have been found so far, namely DP, DO/DZ, DQ and DR, presumably arranged in this order on the chromosome (21). The DP region, the most centromeric one, contains 2 pairs of α and β genes namely SX_α-SX_β and DP_α-DP_β. Most probably the former ones are pseudogenes so that only the latter ones are expressed carrying the known cellularly defined DP allo-specificities (23). Similarly the DQ region encodes respectively DX_α-DX_β and DQ_α-DQ_β genes. Although both pairs of genes may be expressed, only the DQ products expressing the currently known DQ(w1-3) allodeterminants seem to have been identified thus far whereas the situation for DX is not completely known yet (24). The DR gene cluster contains one α and three β genes, one of which is a pseudogene (25). Besides expressing the serologically defined allelic DR antigens (1-w14) these β chains also carry the supertypic DRw52 and DRw53 allospecificities. Furthermore, these chains express – or at least contribute to the expression of – the cellularly defined HLA-D specificities (26). The DO/DZ cluster finally may contain at least two genes, DO_β (27) and DZ_α (28). It has not been established whether these latter genes can actually be expressed or not. The order of the different class II subregions has recently been established

(29). There may be some additional α and β genes which have not yet been detected. An additional level of complexity is that among different haplotypes the number of genes may vary, especially in the DR_β region (30,31).

The expression and extent of allelic polymorphism varies between the different groups of class II genes. Whereas the DP_α, DP_β, DX_α and DX_β genes display a limited polymorphism, the DQ_α and DQ_β ones presumably are very polymorphic. In the DR region, the polymorphism is expressed entirely by the β chains since the α chain is essentially invariant (reviewed in 19-22). Preliminary evidence for DO/DZ_α polymorphism has been suggested (32), whereas nothing is known as yet about DO_β. The polymorphism of the class II molecules is mainly expressed in the NH_2-terminal domains of the respective α and/or β chains (19-22).

The combination of α and β chains leading to the expression of a class II heterodimer is usually restricted to chains coded by the mentioned paired genes of one haplotype. The expressed polymorphism however can be greatly enhanced by cis- or trans-complementation. The cis-complementation of class II chains has recently been described in mice (33) whereas trans-complementary events occur in humans as well (34). Presently, it is not clear to which extent such mechanisms contribute to the generation of additional polymorphism. Recent gene transfection studies in mice have suggested that the pairing of I-Aα and β chains from different haplotypes results in a very low expression on the cell surface in contrast to haplotype identical chains, arguing against trans-complementation as an important mechanism in the generation of such polymorphism (35).

The class I and II molecules are glycosylated prior to their expression on the cell surface. Class I α chains and class II β chains each carry one carbohydrate group, class II α chains two (19). Class II antigens are associated with an invariant or γ chain (M_r: 31K) before but not after expression on the cell surface (36). The function of this chain is unknown but may be related to biosynthesis and transport of α and β chains to the cell surface.

Relatively little is known about the regulation of the expression of class I and class II molecules. Whereas HLA class I molecules are expressed on virtually all nucleated cells as mentioned, in contrast class II antigens are expressed primarily on immunocompetent cells namely B cells, activated T cells and antigen presenting cells (APC) such as monocytes, macrophages, dendritic cells and Langerhans cells. It has been shown however that many (if not in the end it will turn out to be all) other cell lineages can be induced to express these molecules. For instance, class II antigens can also be expressed on hematopoietic progenitor cells (37,38), endothelial cells (39), intestinal epithelial cells (40), keratinocytes (41), thyroid cells (42), astrocytes (43), fibroblasts (44) and so on. In a number of these cases, class II expression was induced or enhanced by γ-interferon (39,42,44,45). On the other hand, substances like prostaglandin (46) may down-regulate class II expression. Besides such soluble factors released by immune or other cells, a gene that regulates class II expression has recently been mapped outside the HLA region. A defect in this gene resulted in a global defect in class II expression (47,48).

The HLA and the H-2 genes and molecules show extensive homologies, not only with regard to the constant regions but also with respect to the polymorphic ones. The H-2 system encoded by chromosome 17 contains three "classical" class I genes (H-2K, H-2D and H-2L) and eight known class II (H-2I) genes ($A_{\beta 3}$, $A_{\beta 2}$, $A_{\beta 1}$, A_α, $E_{\beta 2}$, $E_{\beta 1}$, E_α and $E_{\beta 3}$ arranged in this order on the chromosome, the $A_{\beta 3}$ being the most centromeric one (22)). K, D and L show the most homology with HLA-A, -B and -C respectively (49), $A_{\beta 3}$ with DP, $A_{\beta 2}$ with DO_β (27), $A_{\beta 1}$ and A_α with DQ and finally $E_{\beta (1,2)}$ and E_α with DR.

Besides the discussed class I and class II regions, another region, which has been called class IV, has been mapped telomeric of the HLA-A and H-2D, L region. Molecular genetic analyses of the H-2 class I genes have revealed the existence of a surprising number (20-40) of additional class I like genes per haplotype, besides K, D and L (50,51), which all mapped into the class IV region. Two major subregions were distinguished namely Qa and Tla, which contain most of these genes. Some products of these subregions have been identified. The very limited polymorphism of these products however – in contrast to that of the K, D and L molecules – probably hinders the generation of adequate serological reagents specifically defining these products. In addition, recent evidence suggests that a number of these class I-like genes in fact are pseudogenes and that they may act as donor genes for the exchange information with other class I (like) genes (reviewed in 52). In humans, two such class IV products have been found, namely HT (53) and TCA (54,55). The function of class IV molecules is unknown, but may be related to their primary expression on hematopoietic and tumour cells.

II. MHC class II resticted antigen specific T lymphocyte activation

Unlike B cells, T cells do not respond to free antigen, but only to antigen that is presented to the T cell in association with a MHC molecule. This MHC restriction of T cell activation was first demonstrated in animal models: murine cytotoxic T cells (Tc) specifically lysing autologous lymphocytic choriomeningitis virus (LCM) infected target cells could only lyse similarly infected allogeneic target cells if the latter expressed the same H-2 haplotype (56). In analogy, histocompatible macrophages and T lymphocytes were required in order for antigen to induce T lymphocyte proliferate responses (57). The *in vivo* relevance of MHC restricted T cell responses subsequently was demonstrated in transfer experiments (58,59).

As a rule, Tc are restricted by self class I molecules, whereas helper T cells (Th) are restricted by self class II molecules (60). Here, we will focus only on Th cell responsiveness since it is mainly this type of T cells which is responsible for the induction of protective immunity as well as delayed type hypersensitivity (DTH) reactivity versus *Mycobacterium leprae* in leprosy patients and healthy individuals (61) and thus the subject of our studies. These *M. leprae* reactive

Th cells most probably mediate the activation of macrophages, which is of importance for the intracellular killing of *M. leprae* bacilli (61). Thus far, a major role for Tc cells in the immune response to *M. leprae* has not been suggested by the available data whereas humoral immune responsiveness does not correlate with protective immunity against *M. leprae* (and related mycobacteria) (61; vide infra). (For extensive reviews on MHC and T cell activation the reader may be referred to references 60,62 and 63).

Despite detailed information available on antigenic determinants, polymorphic MHC class II restriction determinants and T cell antigen/MHC receptors which are the essential constituents for the induction of T cell activation, the actual molecular mechanisms leading to T cell activation have remained controversial and unresolved. The main reason beyond doubt is the intricate complexity leading to the formation of the supposed ternary antigen – MHC – T cell receptor complex (62). Each of these three components will be discussed in brief here.

A. Antigen-processing and antigenic determinants

Several studies have suggested that antigen has to be handled or "processed" by APC before it can be presented properly to T cells (reviewed in 64). Antigen would be internalized by the APC, partially degraded in low-pH compartments by a metabolically active process and then recycled to the cell surface as an immunogenic fragment (64). The supposed internal degradation of antigen can be inhibited by lysosomotropic drugs such as chloroquine and NH_4Cl, which are thought to increase the pH and thus to prevent enzymatic degradation, or similarly by protease inhibitors like monensin (65,66). Although the actual internalization of antigen in order for processing to occur lacks formal proof, direct evidence for enzymatic cleavage of antigen, leading to the formation of immunogenic fragments, came from studies in which glutaraldehyde fixed and thus metabolically inactive APC could present *in vitro* trypsinized but not native ovalbumine (67). Thus, fragmentation of antigen was not only necessary but also sufficient to account for antigen processing in these and other studies (see 66). For other antigens, e.g. myoglobin, the mere unfolding rather than degradation of the protein was sufficient for the exposure of apparently internally buried antigenic determinants (68). Besides degradation and/or unfolding of the molecule, other parts of the antigen have to be critically preserved, since for instance the cleavage of helical structures may result in the loss of subsequent T cell responses in some cases (69,70). In other cases antigen processing may not even be necessary at all since native antigen coupled to class II carrying liposomes can induce T cell responses (71). Thus, whereas some antigens may have to be "processed" before being immunogenic for T cells, other antigens might lack that requirement. The processing requirements for different T cell clones may also well be different (72,73).

An interesting observation is that several T cell stimulatory antigenic fragments possess an amphipathic nature, consisting of a non-polar and a polar site (64,74-76). It may well be that the hydrophobic part plays a role in anchoring the peptide to the APC membrane whereas the hydrophilic residues are involved in the stimulation of the antigen/MHC receptor of the T cell. On this basis it seems possible to predict to some extent the T cell stimulatory sites on an antigen (76).

Distinct sites on antigens have been postulated such as the agretope (*antigen recognition*), the site on the antigen which would contact the class II molecule and the epitope, the site that would be seen by the T cell receptor (vide infra). Not all sites of an antigen are primarily immunogenic in that they can activate T cells: immune responses are focussed to relatively limited epitopes on the antigen (77,78). These epitopes are recognized by T cells in a hierarchic manner. This so called "epitope hierarchy" may be dependent also on non-antigenic factor such as the available MHC class II molecules and the available functional T cell repertoire. The mentioned epitope hierarchy can be bypassed by manipulating the antigen (e.g. 77,79) so that T cell responses can be induced against "low-ranked" epitopes. Besides Th antigenic determinants presumably also suppressor determinants can be expressed by antigens (77,79-81). Such epitopes may activate Ts which may down-regulate or abolish antigen induced responses. The presence and/or the relative position in the total "epitope hierarchy" of such suppressor epitopes may influence the final outcome of the immune response.

B. MHC class II expression by APC

The expression of compatible class II molecules is a conditio sine qua non for Th cell activation as pointed out earlier. The quantitative expression of these molecules correlates with the strength of the subsequent T cell response (82-84), and can be modulated by distinct factors such as γ-interferon and prostaglandins (vide supra). The sites on the class II molecules that carry the restriction determinants (RDs) are the polymorphic domains. The comparisons of nucleotide c.q. amino acid sequences of these domains with the patterns of antigen induced Th responses (85-87) as well as the transfection of class II genes into class II negative cells (88) have revealed that a relatively small number of residues actually is involved in the expression of RDs. The substitution of a single residue can result in the complete loss of Th cell responsiveness (87). Transfection studies and the chemical construction of lipid membranes substituted only with purified class II molecules (71,89) have demonstrated that in the presence of the proper antigenic fragment the expression of class II molecules is necessary as well as sufficient for the activation of T cell clones and hybridomas (note that such T cells may be highly selected for independency of other growth factors or counter structures (vide infra)).

Whereas APC originally were thought to be confined to cells such as monocytes, macrophages, dendritic cells, Langerhans cells and Kupffer cells, recently an impressive number of papers appeared in the literature that described other cells which also expressed class II and were capable of presenting antigens to T cells. One group of such cells are B cells, both normal (90) and tumour line derived (91) as well as Epstein-Barr virus transformed ones (EBV-BC) (e.g. 92: see figure 2). The capacity of B cells to present antigen to T cells may be important in the amplification of *in vivo* immune responses. Other cells that can present antigen to T cells include e.g. endothelial cells (93), fibroblasts (94), thyrocytes (95), astrocytes (43), large granular lympho-

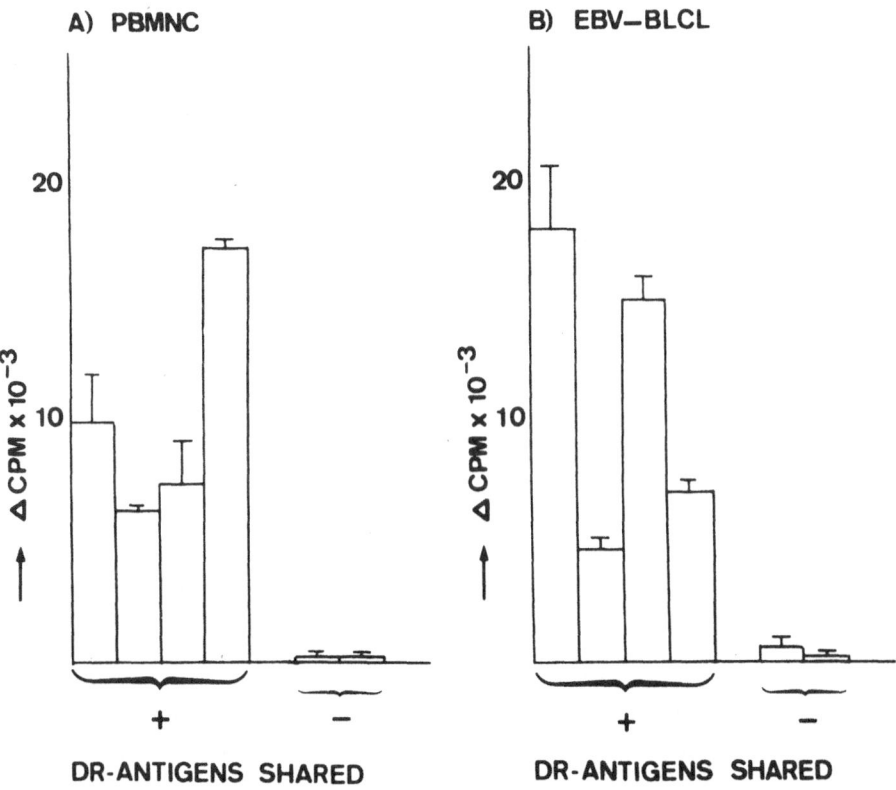

Fig. 2

Presentation of *M. leprae* antigens to T cells by respectively peripheral blood mononuclear cells (PBMNC) (A) and EBV-BC (B) as source of allogeneic APC. The APC either shared (+) or did not share (–) HLA-DR antigens with the *M. leprae* reactive T cell line that had been derived from a tuberculoid leprosy patient. The PBMNC and EBV-BC tested had been derived from the same donors. Each T cell-APC combination is represented by one column. Results are expressed as Δcpmx10^{-3} ± SEM of triplicate cultures. The data were taken from ref. 92.

cytes (96) and activated T cells (97). It may well be that in fact virtually all types of cells can act as APC provided that they can be triggered to express class II antigens. The absence of class II on normal tissue cells may be important for the maintenance of self tolerance. This supposition is inferred from studies in e.g. human thyroiditis, where thyrocytes were found to express HLA-DR presumably as a consequence of γ-interferon stimulation (98). Expression of DR was suggested to endow these cells with the property of presenting auto-antigens to T cells resulting in auto-immunity. Similar observations have been made in other diseases as well (99).

On the other hand, it cannot be inferred that class II positive cells can present antigen to any T cell. For instance, unprimed or resting memory Th cells may only be (re)activated by dendritic cells and not e.g. by macrophages (100). Furthermore, the production of interleukin-1 (IL-1) by APC may be critical for most T cells, although (*in vitro*) cloned and already activated T cells may well have become IL-1 independent. (IL-1 is a multifunctional polypeptide that is produced amongst others by activated macrophages and is involved in T cell stimulation as a T cell differentiation/activation signal apart from antigen/MHC. IL-1 may be released or expressed on the membranes of APC. For a review, the reader may be referred to reference 101).

Furthermore, APC dependent differences in the expression of relevant counter structures for the presumably functional T cell surface antigens such as CD4 (T4/leu 3), CD8 (T8/leu2) and CDw18 (LFA-1) may determine whether a T cell response will occur or not. This may be the explanation why the transfection of MHC genes not always leads to functional antigen presenting transfectants (102).

It is interesting that the nature of the antigen may determine the class II RDs that are used by Th cells (or vice versa). For instance, in mice responses against poly(Glu-Lys-Phe), poly (Glu-Lys-Leu) and pigeon cytochrome c are typically I-E restricted (103,104) whereas antigens like ovalbumin, beef insulin and H-Y induce I-A restricted responses (e.g. 67,82,105,106). Even for only one antigenic molecule, such as myoglobin, that can be presented in association with I-A or I-E, the immunodominance of a given antigenic determinant depended strongly on the restriction element used (107). In man, T cell responses may be restricted predominantly by DR molecules (e.g. figure 3; chapters 5 and 6), but responsiveness against mannan (108) may be typically DQ restricted. In other models, I-A may restrict helper and I-E suppressor T cells as in the case of lactate dehydrogenase (LDH$_\beta$) (106). Similarly, DQ may preferentially restrict antigen specific Ts cells and DR antigen specific Th cells such as in the case of streptococcal cell wall antigens (109).

It recently has become clear that MHC class II molecules can physically interact with antigen, during or before T cell activation. (Interactions between MHC class I antigens and virus (110), penicillin and other drugs (111) and neuropeptides (111) were well known already). The first evidence came from competitive inhibition studies in which T cell responses against certain antigens

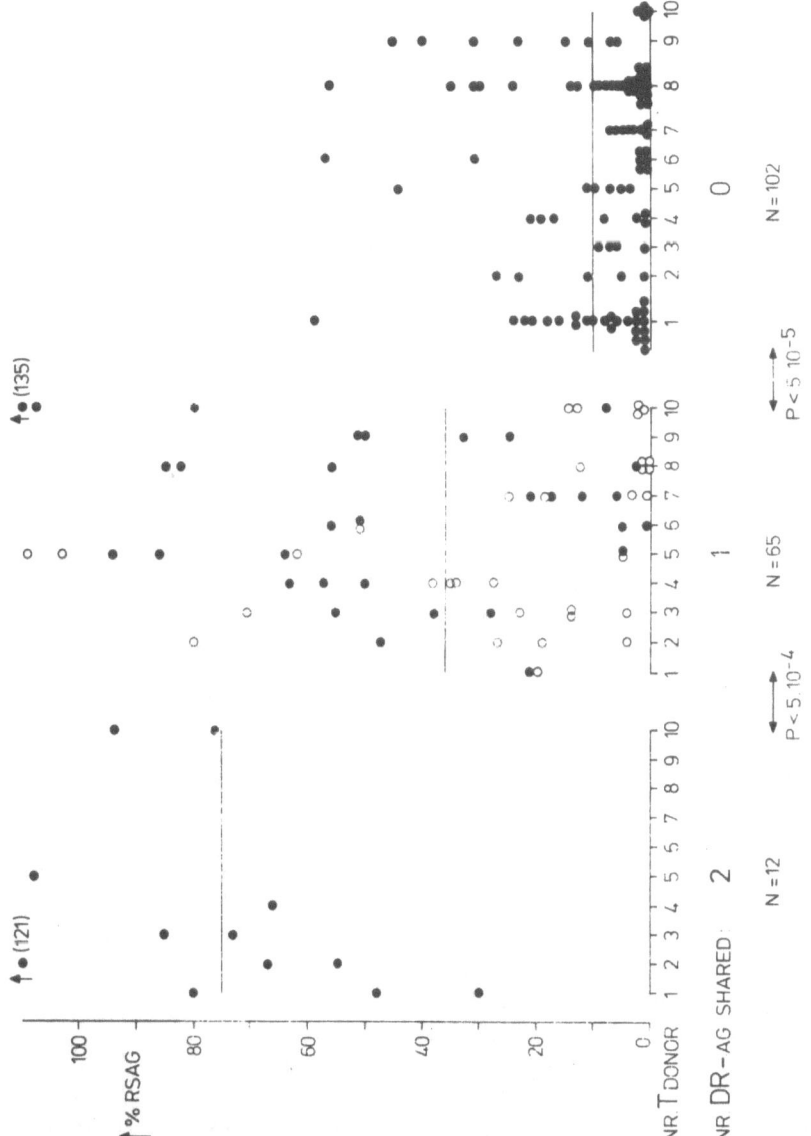

Fig. 3

HLA-DR restriction of PPD and tetanus toxoid specific T cell responses in 179 allogeneic T cell-APC combinations in which respectively 2, 1 or no DR antigens were shared between T cell and APC. In each of the 3 columns, the results for the 10 tested T cell lines derived from 10 different donors are indicated by corresponding numbers. The results are expressed in %RSAG (see also chapter 6). Mean values and significance of the differences between the 3 columns are given. The data are taken from ref. 319.

could be blocked completely by structurally homologous but non-immunogenic antigens (112). This inhibition was antigen and haplotype specific and was explained by competitive binding of the structural homologues to similar or closely related class II epitopes (112-115). Additional evidence for such a physical class II-antigen interaction was provided by the experiments of Heber-Katz *et al.* which suggested that the class II molecule on the APC influenced directly or indirectly the antigen specificity as well as the immune response phenotype of the T cell (116,117). More direct evidence came from studies measuring the binding of antigens to free class II molecules directly (118,119) or indirectly (120,121). Other studies have demonstrated that processed antigen fragments may associate with class II molecules, thus creating immunogenic complexes for T cells (122). Thus direct physical antigen – class II interactions may take place and be relevant for the induction of T cell responses.

C. Antigen/MHC class II recognition by the Th cell

Being once elusive, the receptor for antigen and MHC expressed by T cells has now been identified. After a decade of experimental work (reviewed in 123), two elegant approaches appeared to be successful namely the generation of clonotypic monoclonal antibodies and the isolation of T cell specific messenger-RNA by subtractive hybridization.

Clonotypic antibodies, which specifically react with a particular T cell clone displaying a certain antigen/MHC specificity, can selectively inhibit the function of that clone (124). When these antibodies are made polyvalent by coupling them to a matrix, they can activate specifically these same T cells (125). These antibodies can precipitate a heterodimeric glycoprotein complex from the cell surface of the relevant but not of another T cell clone. This complex consists of two chains, α and β respectively, with M_r's of 45-50 K and 40 K (in mice both chains have a M_r of about 43 K) (123). Both chains possess variable and constant regions and are connected by a disulfide bond, whereas also intrachain disulfide bonds are present.

The second approach, namely the isolation of T cell clone specific mRNA by subtractive hybridization led to the identification of the genes encoding the T cell receptor glycoproteins (126,127). The genes coding for the α chain consist of several segments encoding multiple V(variable), D(diversity), J(joining) and C(constant) regions and those for the β chain of V, J and C regions (123). Rearrangment of these separate segments leads to the formation of functional genes. Besides the α and β genes, a third closely related family of genes, called γ, has been described (128). Like α and β genes, γ genes can rearrange, at least in some T cells. Only very recently a product of this latter group of genes has probably been identified (129,130). The protein structure predicted from the α and β sequences suggests the presence of two disulfide bonded domains in each chain expressed on the outer cell surface, as well as the presence of a transmembranic region and a cytoplasmic tail (123).

Although the mentioned inhibition studies with clonotypic antibodies already suggested that this single molecular complex was involved in the antigen/MHC recognition by the T cell, so far the most straightforward answer has come from experiments in which the α and β T cell receptor genes of one murine T cell clone were transfected into another one with a distinct specificity. The results indicated that the recipient T cell was endowed with the antigen/MHC specificity of the donor T cell, thus strongly suggesting that the α and β chains are essential and sufficient for MHC restricted antigen recognition (131).

The T cell antigen/MHC receptor is physically associated with the T3 complex in humans. This complex consists of three chains: $\gamma(M_r$: 25 K), $\delta(M_r$: 20 K) and $\epsilon(M_r$: 20K) (132) (not to be mixed up with the putative T cell receptor γ and δ proteins). In mice, a similar T3 like protein complex exists (133). Surface expression of the antigen/MHC receptor – T3 complex requires the presence of all compounds. The singular expression of either T3 or the antigen/MHC receptor has not been observed so far (123) although on selected T cells which do not express the T cell receptor α, β chains but (instead?) the putative γ and δ chains, T3 expression was observed in close association with these γ and δ products (129,130). Anti-T3 antibodies often coprecipitate the α and β chains and – like clonotypic antibodies – can inhibit or induce T cell activation, dependent on the experimental conditions used (123).

Little is known about how the T cell receptor actually recognizes antigen/MHC. No simple correlations were found between antigen and/or MHC specificity and α and β chain variability although one report claimed that changes in one (β) chain may somehow alter the MHC specificity without significantly affecting the antigen specificity of a T cell (134). Although the original dispute about whether a single receptor or whether two independent receptors are responsible for antigen/MHC recognition seems to have ended in favour of the single receptor model (63) nevertheless it is not resolved yet whether two distinct sites (two combining site model) or rather one single site (single combining site model) on the receptor recognize(s) antigen/MHC. In addition it is not completely clear what part of the antigen/MHC complex is recognized by the T cell receptor. In principle this could vary from the extreme forms such as altered epitopes on the MHC part (altered self) or altered epitopes on the antigen (altered antigen) as a consequence of the interaction between both parts to intermediate models which would propose the simultaneous recognition of parts of both components (reviewed in 63).

The role of the thymus in the selection of the T cell repertoire is beyond the scope of this review. It is generally accepted that the thymus imposes tolerance to self antigens on T cells differentiating within the thymus (135). Secondly, the thymus determines the MHC class II restriction repertoire as well as the Ir phenotype of such T cells (136). For an extensive review on these subjects the reader may be refered to reference 137.

Besides the T cell antigen/MHC clonotypic receptor also other non-clonotypic T cell activation pathways exist apart from the T3 complex. One such an alternative pathway is via the CD2 or T11 T cell specific molecule, the sheep red blood cell receptor, which expresses distinct functional epitopes (138). Another one is via the 9.3 (T90/44) antigen, a 90K homodimer (139). The physiological relevance and ligands of these 2 structures are unknown, although T11 may be the receptor for "interleukin-4A", a growth factor produced by activated T cells that can induce antigen independent proliferation in resting T cell populations (140). In addition, T cells can be triggered by mitogens and phorbol esters as well (141). The mechanism and putative receptors for these agents are unknown although the mitogen phytohaemagglutinin (PHA) may use the CD2 molecules as receptors (142).

All pathways culminate in a rapid increase in intracytoplasmatic free Ca^{2+}, one of the first events upon receptor triggering (141) and finally in the production of interleukin-2 (IL-2) and the expression of IL-2 receptors. IL-2 enhances T cell expansion but also influences B cell growth and differentiation (143). In addition, other factors are produced such as γ-interferon, a major macrophage activating factor (144), B cell growth and B cell differentiation factor.

Although the specificity of T cell activation depends on the above discussed T cell antigen/MHC receptor, additional molecules may play a role as stabilizing or adhesion structures during antigen dependent T cell activation. For Th, one such a structure may be the CD4 antigen (T4/leu3) (in the mouse: L3T4) that is expressed mainly on helper/ inducer T cells and class II specific alloproliferative and/or cytotoxic T cells. Anti CD4 antibodies are able to block Th cell activation. From the finding that the T cell response induced by transfected class II and antigen could be blocked by CD4 antibodies, it was concluded that the CD4 molecule binds to the class II molecule on the APC (145). However, recent evidence suggests that anti CD4 antibodies may also transduce a negative signal, rendering the T cell unresponsive to subsequent antigen specific triggering (146). Other "adhesion" molecules may include LFA-1 (147) and may be additional structures as well.

III. MHC class II Ir genes

A. Ir genes

Interindividual differences in the development of diseases have been noted since ancient medical history. Not until experimental animal models became available however, the influence of genetic versus environmental factors on the immune response could be determined. Probably, many different genes and products are involved in the regulation of immune responses. In principle, all these genes thus can be defined as immune response (Ir) genes. In the case of polymorphism in these Ir genes, the interindividual differences in such genes may give rise to interindividual differences in immunereactivity against certain foreign antigens and consequently may result in differential susceptibility or alternatively resistance to disease induced by pathogens. The polymorphism of Ir genes may be biologically relevant to ensure the integrity of the species in the case of e.g. epidemics caused by lethally infectious microorganisms. Certain individuals with the "incorrect" Ir genes for the particular agent will be at the disadvantage and may die whereas others with the appropriate Ir gene phenotype will be able to generate a protective immune response. Given the presence of Ir genes and their consequences (e.g. nonresponsiveness or hyperresponsiveness both of which can lead to disease and death (148,149)), the differential distribution of such genes will spread the risks resulting from genetically determined inappropriate immune responsiveness among the population.

Polymorphic Ir genes may be antigen non-specific or antigen specific. The selective breeding of mice with respectively high and low antibody responses against erythrocyte antigens has revealed the existence of at least 10 independent polymorphic Ir genes (150). These genes however turned out to be mostly antigen non-specific since they controlled high or low responsiveness against a number of unrelated antigens as well. Another example of an antigen non-specific Ir gene is the non H-2-linked control of natural resistance or innate immunity by a gene located on the murine chromosome 1. This gene(s) controls natural resistance against a series of intracellular micro-organisms such as *M. bovis, L. monocytogenes, S. typhimurium, M. lepraemurium* etc. (151,152).

B. MHC Ir genes

Antigen specific Ir genes were discovered first when guinea pigs were immunized with synthetic antigens such as dinitrophenyl-poly-L-lysine (DNP-PLL) and polymers of glutamic acid and lysine (GL). It appeared that animals could be divided into responders and nonresponders to these antigens (153). From subsequent breeding experiments it was concluded that a single autosomal dominant gene was responsible for this dichotomy in responsiveness, and that the effect was antigen specific since responses against unrelated antigens were not influenced. Similar observations were made in mice immunized with another synthetic antigen ((T,G)-A-L), and it was there that this antigen specific Ir gene was found to be linked with H-2 genes and – later – to map into the H-2I region (154). The principle of this approach, i.e. the study of antigen specific immune responses against antigens with a highly restricted number of immunogenic sites (namely synthetic repetitive antigenic polymers or alloantigens differing in few regions from autoantigens such as insulin, cytochrome C, lysozyme, myoglobin) allowed the detection of MHC class II linked antigen specific Ir genes in several different species (63).

However, MHC (class I and class II) Ir genes in fact are of more importance than providing elegant models for devoted scientists who are studying genetically controlled differences in responsiveness against highly selected or synthetic antigens that an animal may perhaps never encounter *in vivo*. The studies of Lilly *et al.* (155) indicated that Gross leukemia virus infections were lethal only in $H-2^k$ but not in $H-2^b$ or F_1 mice, thus suggesting a role for MHC linked genes in susceptibility or resistance to infection. Later studies showed that e.g. $H-2D^q$ mice died of high Tc responsiveness against LCM-virus (148) whereas $H-2K^{bm1}$ mutant mice died at a lower virus dose as a consequence of Tc non-responsiveness against Sendai virus (149). Another example is that acquired immunity against *L. monocytogenes* in (naturally) susceptible mice is controlled by H-2 genes (156) as is the formation of granulomata upon infection with *M. lepraemurium* (157). These and numerous other studies have clearly established the importance of MHC Ir genes in the control of the immune response against pathogenic micro-organisms, and in the control of susceptibility or resistance to the development of disease.

MHC class II Ir genes control mainly T cell dependent antigen specific immune responses (reviewed in 63,158). Although this observation was made consistently and frequently, the site of Ir gene expression remained unclear at first (63). By now it has been clearly established that the products of MHC class II Ir genes are the MHC class II molecules themselves. The overwhelming body of evidence in support of this notion included: (i) the striking parallels existing between Ir gene- and MHC class II restriction phenomena (63), (ii) the ability to inhibit T cell proliferative responses against antigens under Ir gene control with anti class II (monoclonal) antibodies (e.g. 159,160) (iii) similarly, the ability to inhibit antigen specific suppression by anti class II subgroup (I-E) specific antibodies, thus presumably blocking I-E restricted antigen specific Ts cells and revealing latent responsiveness (106), (iv) the finding that transgenic mice, that had been created by the transfection of I-Eα genes into fertilized eggs of mice strains which do not express I-E molecules as a consequence of an Eα related genomic deletion, not only could express I-E molecules but also simultaneously had regained responsiveness against typically I-E restricted antigens such as poly (Glu-Lys-Phe) (103,104).

Thus, at least in experimental animals the products of MHC class II Ir genes are the MHC class II molecules. The same applies to MHC class I Ir genes and class I molecules (see e.g. 148,149). (some non-MHC antigen specific Ir genes have been identified as well (e.g. 161) whereas one non-MHC locus (162) can code for helper T cell restriction determinants, but these findings represent exceptions).

C. Mechanisms of MHC class II Ir genes

Although it is clear that MHC class II Ir genes determine the way in which T cells see antigen, the precise mechanisms of the Ir gene controlled T cell (non) responsiveness are not completely clear yet. Different models have been proposed (vide infra) in order to explain such antigen specific Ir gene effects. Initially, strong arguments pro or contra one or another mechanism were put forward. However, at present it seems that these models are not a priori mutually exclusive and that – dependent on the antigen and Ir gene involved – one or another model may provide the right explanation for the observed phenomenon.

Basically, three types of models have been developed. The first type of models assumes that there is a so-called "hole" or "gap" in the T cell repertoire, leading to a lack of T cells capable of responding to certain antigen/MHC class II complexes (163,164). Presumably, multiple mechanisms can create such holes in the T cell repertoire for instance the deletion or inactivation of certain T cell populations (165) or the failure to positively select T cells. The second type of models assumes a defect at the level of the antigen presenting cell, such as a defect in the processing machinery, or – more specifically – the inability of class II molecules to create an immunogenic complex together with antigen for T cells (118,166). The third type of models postulates the preferential activation of antigen/class II specific Ts cells, which could also cause specific unresponsiveness (76,79,106). Especially in the case of multiple antigenic determinants present on the antigen such as in the case of micro-organisms antigen specific suppression may be an easier explanation for non-responsiveness than the creation of multiple holes in the T cell repertoire.

Whereas these models as mentioned initially tried to account for antigen specific non- or low-responsiveness, they may also partly explain high responsiveness against foreign antigens, or responsiveness to auto-antigens. One example may be the $H-2D^q$ associated high Tc responsiveness against LCM virus, resulting in brain damage and death (148). Another example may be experimental allergic encephalomyelitis (EAE) which can be induced in MHC susceptible animals upon immunization with myelin basic protein (MBP), resulting in auto-reactive MBP specific class II restricted T cells that mediate the disease (167).

D. Evidence for human Ir genes

Although these and other experimental animal models have demonstrated the presence of MHC class II Ir genes as well as revealed in part their mode of action in the control of Th responsiveness, relatively limited evidence for such Ir genes is available in human models. Obvious limitations in the search for human Ir genes are, besides ethical ones, the lack of congenic and recombinant individuals, hampering the assessment of the influence of single genes or genomic regions on immune responses. Thus, one has to take advantage of naturally occurring immunologically relevant phenomona, such as infectious and auto-immune diseases, and responses to defined antigens upon primary immunizations.

Following the line along which animal Ir genes were discovered, namely the use of simple synthetic antigenic determinants, human Ir genes were mapped into the HLA region for (H,G)-A-L and (T,G)-A-L (168). Similarly, a number of HLA related (mainly *in vitro*) differences in immune responses to defined (microbial or other) antigens were found such as for mumps virus and several fungi (169), streptococcal antigen (169-173), influenza A (174), vaccinia virus (175), tetanus toxoid (176), *Schistosoma japonicum* antigens (177), short ragweed pollen antigen (178), *Salmonella adelaide* (179), cedar pollen antigen (180), measles (181), (T,G)-A-L (182), mycobacterial antigens (183), herpes simplex virus (184), malaria (185), Epstein-Barr virus (186). The *in vivo* relevance of these *in vitro* observed interindividual differences in immune responsiveness in relation to susceptibility or resistance to disease could not be resolved entirely, probably with the exception of cedar pollen antigen, schistosomal antigen and mycobacteria where a relationship between the observed *in vitro* differences in immune responsiveness and disease has been postulated. Indeed, the first two studies suggested that HLA linked Is genes (with respectively DR5DQw3 and Dw12DQw1) control immune responsiveness and thus possibly suscep- tibility to disease and proposed that the HLA class II molecules might well be the actual products of these class II linked Is genes (187). Evidence for DR3 restricted low responsiveness of T cells from tuberculoid leprosy patients activated with *M. leprae* antigen in the presence of allogeneic monocytes has been collected in a population where DR3 was associated with that same type of leprosy. These results suggested that DR3 molecules may be the products of an Ir gene for *M. leprae* in that population (188,189). Similar evidence that DR3 and DR7 molecules may be the products of an Ir gene for gluten has been presented by Scott *et al.* (190) in celiac disease that is associated with both DR3 and DR7 (191).

Thus, whereas relatively few *in vitro* observed HLA Ir/Is gene effects have an *in vivo* counterpart related to disease, most of them do not. Vice versa, several associations between HLA antigens and diseases triggered by known foreign agents (*in vivo*) have been described, but although in these cases the presence of Ir or Is genes may be expected, more evidence, e.g. from *in vitro* studies, would be necessary before it can be established that the HLA molecules are the Ir/Is products here. Some examples of such diseases are leprosy (vide infra, with the exception of the mentioned study (188)), typhoid and yellow fever (R.R.P. de Vries, personal communication), tuberculosis (192,193), gonorroe (194), syphilis (194), respiratory disease caused by *H. influenza* (195), poliomyelitis (196), ocular histoplasmosis (197), reactive arthropathies follo- wing infection with *S. flexneri, S. dysenteriae, Yersinia enterocolitica*, and several salmonella and campylobacter species (ref. in 198), rubella (199) and malaria (200).

The majority of diseases that are associated with certain HLA alleles thus far consists of diseases with auto-immune characteristics. The fact that the supposed triggering agents for such diseases have remained essentially undefined has severely hampered further studies to their pathogenesis. The recent isolation of organ specific auto-reactive T cells from the thyroid gland in Graves' patients may perhaps represent a new line of research in this mysterious area (201). The associations between HLA and auto-immune diseases have been summarized in great detail elsewhere (191,202) and will not be discussed in this brief review.

Thus, as stated in the beginning of this section, relatively little is known about the nature of human Ir/Is genes. Their existence is likely on the base of experimental work in animals. *In vitro* and/or *in vivo* differences in immune responsiveness related with HLA as well as the many HLA-disease associations certainly support that notion. However, additional studies exploring the mechanisms of HLA-Ir/Is gene controlled immune responsiveness and/or susceptibility or resistance to disease would seem necessary, and could perhaps be carried out preferably in these cases where the etiological antigens have been well characterized. Such studies may provide important answers and clues to clarify other HLA-disease associations. The more precise definition of antigens (e.g. synthetic or recombinant DNA antigen structures) may become helpful by limiting the antigenic determinants involved. The more accurate mapping of HLA genes and products, c.q. gene fragments and epitopes may open up new ways as well in identifying HLA Ir/Is genes. For instance, in type I diabetes mellitus, resistance against the disease is not only associated with DR2 but also with a polymorphic DQ_β genomic fragment of 15 kb (restriction fragment length polymorphism (RFLP)) that probably codes for a monoclonal antibody (TA10) defined DQ epitope (203). In myasthenia gravis, also a 15 kb DQ_β RFLP was found to correlate with susceptibility (204). If for instance the same DQ_β RFLP would confer resistance to type I diabetes but susceptibility to myasthenia gravis, this RFLP could code for a typical HLA Ir gene. Many more of such newly defined Ir/Is gene markers probably will become available in the near future.

An extraordinary immunological disease where HLA linked Ir/Is genes may play a role and which will be discussed in the following section is leprosy. Our studies on the mechanism of HLA Ir/Is genes have focussed on this disease since the antigen *(M. leprae)*, the responsible immune cells (Th cells) and the HLA class II alleles as possible markers for Ir and Is genes are known. The next section will review in brief the immunology of leprosy as well as the role of HLA in leprosy.

IV. HLA and immune responsiveness in leprosy: a model for the study of human MHC Ir and Is genes

A. The leprosy spectrum

Leprosy is a chronic infectious disease which is caused by *Mycobacterium leprae*. It ranks second behind tuberculosis in the order of human diseases caused by mycobacteria, and it afflicts 10-15 million people mainly in developing countries (205). In endemic areas, its prevalence may exceed 1%. Although these numbers may not seem exceedingly high, leprosy is a major problem in the third world, because of the high frequency of severe rest deformities of the distal extremities as well as the strong social stigmatization.

Whereas most individuals who are exposed to *M. leprae* are resistant to the disease and develop an effective immune response to the bacillus, a small percentage of infected individuals will develop the disease (206). Perhaps the most intriguing feature of the disease is the striking interindividual variability in clinical symptoms that will appear in the course of the disease. This variability in clinical manifestations closely parallels the cell mediated immune response (CMI) which is produced by the host against *M. leprae* (61, 206). A number of systematic classifications have been proposed, but so far the most commonly used is that of Ridley and Jopling (207). This classification distinguishes five main groups of leprosy which form the so-called leprosy spectrum: (polar) tuberculoid (TT), borderline tuberculoid (BT), (mid)borderline (BB), borderline lepromatous (BL) and (polar) lepromatous (LL) leprosy. However, before developing one of these more or less defined clusters of symptoms, patients may initially present with one or few ill-defined hypopigmented macules, some sensory loss and histopathologically often nonspecific features. This sixth or indeterminate (I) form of leprosy may regress spontaneously, remain stable for a period of time or proceed to one of the 5 mentioned types of leprosy (61).

In TT leprosy, the "high resistant" form of the disease, one or few macules or raised, usually hypopigmented skin lesions are found with a loss of local sensory function. Quite commonly, one or more of the nerves are thickened and may appear to be damaged and often even destroyed when examined histologically. TT lesions are predominated by highly ordered granulomata which contain epitheloid cells, multinucleated giant cells, and large numbers of T lymphocytes, the majority of which carries the CD4 marker whereas few are CD8 positive (208-212). Few if any bacilli can be detected in these lesions. These patients show high responses to *M. leprae* antigens injected into the skin as well as in *in vitro* T cell proliferation assays and have low antibody titers to *M. leprae* (61,206). On the opposite pole of the leprosy spectrum LL or "low resistant" patients are found. Such patients will – if untreated – develop numerous skin lesions consisting initially of multiple hypopigmented macules and later noduli and large infiltrates, often accompanied by the characteristic enlarged ear lobes and destroyed nasal cartilage and bones. Extensive and diffuse, often symmetrical damage of dermal nerves may lead to progressive anesthesia (61, 206). Numerous bacilli are present, not only in the skin, but also in the peripheral blood, liver, spleen and bone marrow. Histologically, LL lesions consist mainly of undifferentiated macrophages which – in untreated cases – are packed with massive numbers of live and intact bacilli, thus producing their typical foamy appearance. The few T lymphocytes present, which are mainly of the CD8 and not of the CD4 subset, are diffusely spread throughout the lesions with a clearcut lack of organization (208-212). LL patients show a characteristic T cell unresponsiveness towards *M. leprae* antigens in skin testing as well as in *in vitro* T cell stimulation assays, but produce high levels of circulating antibodies against the bacillus (61,206,213). Within the LL type of leprosy, 2 subtypes are usually distinguished namely subpolar LL (LLs) in which still some BL features may be found, and polar LL (LLp). This subdivision of the LL pole may be of importance with respect to the nature of the *M. leprae* unresponsiveness (vide infra).

In between those 2 extremes of the leprosy spectrum various other forms are distinguished which are either more tuberculoid or more lepromatous in character with intermediate symptoms. Thus, the spectrum is continuous. Patients may move from one type to another: in general, untreated patients tend to move to the lepromatous pole whereas treated patients may shift to the tuberculoid one. However, the true polar forms of the disease, TT and LLp, are stable. Thus, the type of leprosy which develops upon infection in susceptible individuals reflects the type of cell mediated immuneresponsiveness of the host against *M. leprae*.

Acute episodes of immunopathological reactions may occur in several of these types of leprosy. Such acute episodes are divided into type 1 leprosy reactions which may be subdivided in upgrading or reversal reactions and downgrading reactions, and type 2 leprosy reactions, synonymous to erythema nodosum leprosum (ENL). Reversal reactions can affect in principle all borderline (BT-BL) patients. They are characterized by sudden clinical changes representing a shift to the tuberculoid pole of the spectrum, a rapid increase in CMI to *M. leprae*, and often acute neuritis episodes, that may lead to profound and irreversible nerve damage (214). Reversal reactions commonly occur in the first year of anti-leprosy treatment. The etiology is not known, as is the case with downgrading reactions, that in contrast are associated with a shift to the lepromatous pole, and occur mainly in untreated borderline cases. ENL appears in subjects with BL-LL leprosy where the CMI against *M. leprae* is weak or absent but high levels of antibodies to *M. leprae* exist. It presents as nodular erythematous lesions characterized by polynuclear infiltrates and granular deposits of IgG and C3, and may become systemic, presumably as a consequence of circulating immune complexes (215).

As mentioned, nerve damage is a frequent complication of leprosy, occurring along the whole spectrum. However, the nature of nerve damage in the tuberculoid and the lepromatous parts of the spectrum is quite different. In TT leprosy, nerve destruction in itself is often severe, but localized to a relatively small area. Nerve damage per se in BT leprosy may be less severe, but due to the larger dissemination of the disease and the more frequent involvement of larger nerves, the overall damage may be much worse for the patient, and result in chronic disabilities (61,214). The real nature of nerve damage in the tuberculoid types of leprosy is not clear, but seems to be closely associated with strong and/or increased CMI to *M. leprae*. For instance, during reversal reactions an acute increase of CMI against *M. leprae* has been reported (216). The nerves become embedded in epitheloid cell-lymphocytic (CD4$^+$) infiltrates that may invade and finally even completely replace nearby nerves. Similar observations with regard to a role for T cell mediated immunity in nerve damage have been made in experimental mice, where the grafting of syngeneic thymus tissue into *M. leprae* infected thymectomized lepromatous-like animals could produce tuberculoid-like nerve damage (217). In other experiments, bystander demyelination developed as a consequence of strong CMI towards injected foreign antigens in the neigbourhood of nerve tissue (218). Injection of animals with peripheral nerve antigens could produce tuberculoid leprosy like skin lesions (219-221).

A different type of nerve damage is observed at the lepromatous pole: slow but steadily progressive and disseminated damage occurs, predominantly in the cutaneous nerves. *M. leprae* bacilli display a remarkable preference to invade Schwann cells and other endoneural and perineural cells including macrophages. Large numbers of bacilli may accumulate there. The consequent thickening of the epineurium and demyelination leads to gradual deterioration of the involved nerves (61,215). How and why the bacilli invade Schwann cells is poorly understood. Since such cells presumably are not active in the intracellular killing of bacilli, and are not known to express class II molecules they may provide immunologically priviliged sites for *M. leprae*, protecting it from being recognized by T cells (222).

B. The leprosy bacillus

Mycobacterium leprae was the first human pathogenic bacillus which was discovered, as described by Armauer Hansen in 1874 (223). The study of this acid fast bacillus has been hampered severely by the fact that it cannot be grown in *in vitro* cultures. Although *M. leprae* bacilli have been observed to incorporate some ^{3}H-thymidine and to increase in number when cultured within macrophages (224), these procedures do not allow the harvesting of large numbers of organisms. A first breakthrough in this respect was the observation of Shepard that *M. leprae* can be grown in the mouse footpad, albeit to a limited ($\pm$ 10^6 bacilli) extent (225). T cell deficient mice can deliver up to 10^8 organisms. A second breakthrough came with the finding that the nine-banded armadillo (*Dasypus novemcinctus*) is susceptible to infection with *M. leprae* (226). Once injected with live bacilli, the infection spreads throughout the body and finally can result in the presence of 10^{12} viable bacilli per gram of liver and spleen tissue. At present, these armadillos are the main source of leprosy bacilli. Recently, it was shown that the grey mangabey monkey is susceptible to leprosy as well (227). A third and major breakthrough was realized recently when the genome of the leprosy bacillus was cloned and expressed in *Escherichia coli* (228). Thus for the first time an unlimited source of well defined antigens has become available (vide infra).

The leprosy bacillus is generally classified as belonging to the mycobacterial species, being acid-fast and containing mycobacterial high molecular weight mycolic acids, cross-linked peptidoglycans and arabinogalactan (229). Studies with monoclonal antibodies have revealed the existence of relatively few *M. leprae* specific protein epitopes. These epitopes are carried by proteins with M_r's of 12, 18, 28, 36 and 64K (230). An additional antibody defined specific epitope(s) is carried by the *M. leprae* phenolic glycolipid-I, the terminal trisaccharide of which is essentially required for recognition by both monoclonal antibodies and serum antibodies (230,231). These latter antibodies, present in sera of mainly lepromatous patients as well as presumably susceptible contacts, provide an important tool for serodiagnostic purposes (231). Most other antibody defined epitopes are shared with few till many other mycobacteria (230).

Although T cell mediated immunity is of primary importance for protective immunity, DTH reactivity (often but not always correlating with the former) and maybe immunopathology at the tuberculoid end of the spectrum, the antigens seen by such T cells have remained ill defined. A soluble *M. leprae* cell wall protein, called MLW-1, has been reported to contain a *M. leprae* specific epitope besides a number of crossreactive ones (232). Animal studies have suggested that crossreactive antigens may induce DTH and protective immunity (233-237). Recently however, cloned *M. leprae* reactive T cells from patients as well as healthy immunized volunteers were isolated that recognized an unexpected high number of *M. leprae* specific epitopes, part of which could be mapped on the mentioned *M. leprae* specific proteins (238, chapter 3). These data may indicate that in humans these *M. leprae* specific epitopes may be relevant for the induction of effective immunity. This may explain in part the generally disappointing protective effect of BCG vaccination trials in Burma, India and Papua New Guinea, the only encouraging result coming from the Uganda trial (reviewed in 239).

C. Pathogenesis of tuberculoid and lepromatous leprosy

As mentioned in the foregoing section, TT leprosy has several characteristics of high and perhaps even excessive T cell responsiveness against *M. leprae*. This may be underlined by the virtual absence of intact bacilli in tuberculoid lesions, suggesting that the produced immune response not necessarily has only a protective character. The discussed experimental induction of nerve damage by sensitization to nerve antigens and by immune responses against antigens in the proximity of nerves as well as the observed increased CMI towards *M. leprae* during reversal reactions may support that concept. Crossreactivity between mycobacterial antigens and self-components has been described in a number of cases (240,241): antigenic mimicry may lead to a break of tolerance to auto-antigens and therefore true auto-immunity. Another possibility however would be bystander damage as a nonspecific consequence of inflammatory reactions in the proximity of nerves (217). In this respect, the discussed predilection of *M. leprae* for Schwann cells may focus such reactions to the nerves (242). Such a bystander damage may be completely nonspecific, or partly nonspecific. In the latter case e.g. Schwann cells may be destroyed or damaged nonspecifically with subsequent leakage of auto-antigens – normally undetectable for T cells – to class II positive APC which on their turn might trigger auto-immune reactivity.

The most prominent immunological feature of LL leprosy is the *M. leprae* specific (CMI) anergy. Although some reports have claimed decreased immune responsiveness to other antigens as well (243-245) it has been generally accepted that this unresponsiveness is selective for antigens expressed by *M. leprae* (61,206,213). It is intriguing that for instance the CMI against *M. tuberculosis* and BCG in LL leprosy is unaffected (61,213,246) whereas these mycobacteria share a large number of antigenic determinants with *M. leprae*. This paradox has fascinated immunologists for many years. Basically, three types of explanations have been proposed, which parallel those accounting for MHC Ir en Is gene effects (vide supra). First, APC might be deficient in the processing and/or presentation of *M. leprae* antigens to T cells in LL patients. Although two groups have claimed evidence for that (247-249), only few combinations of allogeneic T cells and monocytes have been tested whereas the defective presentation of *M. leprae* by LL monocytes to responder T cells was not controlled for other antigens and in one study could equally be explained by HLA class II mismatching between T cells and APC (247). The majority of the studies, including our own, has shown that LL monocytes or APC can present *M. leprae* to T cells from responder individuals (250,251, chapter 6), excluding an apparent defect on the APC level. A second explanation for the observed *M. leprae* specific anergy has been the deletion or inactivation of *M. leprae* reactive helper T cells (250,252). Whereas indeed the frequency of circulating T cells may be decreased, it would seem rather difficult to conceive how T cells against all – presumably many – antigenic determinants expressed by *M. leprae* could be tolerized or deleted. Furthermore, although still controversial, it has been shown that at least some LL patients can be restored in their T cell responses to *M. leprae* (proliferation or γ-interferon production) by the addition of exogenous IL-2. However, the extent to which these findings can be generalized as well as their actual significance remains the subject of debate (253-260). These studies however provide evidence that circulating T cells reactive with *M. leprae* may exist in at least some LL patients. The conflicting outcomes of these studies may be explained in part by heterogeneity within the lepromatous group, BL and LLs patients being low responders, whereas only LLp patients would be true nonresponders.

The third model to explain the *M. leprae* specific unresponsiveness is the presence of suppressor cells and factors. Whereas on the one hand this model is the most favoured, on the other hand a variety of experimental approaches has produced a large number of results which sometimes are conflicting and not easy to interpret. Furthermore, suppressive influences of *M. leprae* have been noted along the whole spectrum of leprosy as well as in healthy contacts (261-264), thus not explaining the *M. leprae* specific suppression in LL. The most suggestive but indirect evidence for suppression perhaps comes from the mentioned histopathological studies that showed a CD8 positive lymphocyte predominance in LL as opposed to TT lesions (208-212) and *in vivo* and *in vitro* studies where the CMI against other mycobacteria was unimpaired although these latter bacilli share multiple antigenic determinants with *M. leprae* (229).

The main experimental evidence for suppressor cells and factors in LL leprosy can be summarized as follows. Mehra and colleagues observed *M. leprae* mediated suppression of concanavalin (con A) stimulated lymphocytes of LL and borderline but not TT patients or healthy controls (265). Suppressor cells resided mainly in the CD8 (TH2 or OKT8) positive T cell subpopulation but in some cases also adherent cells from LL patients could suppress (266). In a third of the (borderline) lepromatous patients, T cell proliferative responses to *M. leprae* were observed in CD8 depleted but not in unfractionated T cells (267). The same investigators showed later that this T lymphocyte mediated suppression probably was induced by a *M. leprae* specific epitope residing on the terminal trisaccharide of the *M. leprae* phenolic glycolipid-I. Removal of this epitope or blocking with a specific monoclonal antibody abolished the observed suppression (268). At variance with these findings, Nath and colleagues presented a number of experiments showing that *M. leprae* induced peripheral blood suppressor cells were present in TT patients as well, even more pronounced than in LL ones (263). Similar findings were reported using the above mentioned phenolic glycolipid-I (269). Proliferative responses to PPD (purified protein derivative of *M. tuberculosis*) were reduced in the presence of *M. leprae* as well (263). Another study provided evidence for suppressive monocytes in LL but not TT leprosy (249,270). Similar studies in the con A system by a third group confirmed the findings of Nath *et al.* with respect to suppression in TT leprosy and extended this observation to healthy controls in addition (271). A fourth group which had reported on *M. leprae* reactive suppressor cells in healthy controls (264) did not find suppression in HLA-D identical sibling coculture experiments of peripheral blood mononuclear cells (261). A variety of other studies provided evidence for adherent cell- or macrophage mediated suppression in LL leprosy (248,270,272) or deficiencies in these cells (273,274).

Thus, although many workers agree upon the presence of suppressor cells in LL leprosy and in leprosy in general, the reported results are rather divergent. Differences in techniques, antigens, patient populations, stages of disease and possibly suppressor mechanisms may account for at least part of this heterogeneity. Nevertheless, the issue of suppression in LL leprosy and its relevance for the development of this form of the disease (e.g. causative to or a consequence of the development of LL?) remains an intriguing and open one. The recent demonstration of suppressive mechanisms, in the case of other mycobacteria as well may indicate that suppression inducing determinants may not be confined to *M. leprae* only (275), and may be helpful in unravelling the epitopes and mechanisms of mycobacterial antigen induced suppression.

D. HLA and leprosy

In 1841 Simpson stated that "few facts in the history of tubercular leprosy seem to be more universally admitted by all writers on the disease, both ancient and modern, than the transmission of the predisposition to it from parents to offspring" (cited from 276). Almost a century later, this interest in the possible genetic predisposition to leprosy was renewed (277), leading to the study of Spickett (278) who proposed that the type of leprosy was determined by hereditary factors, and that of Beiguelman, reporting an increased concordance for leprosy type within families (279). An important study among monozygotic and dizygotic twins concordant or discordant for leprosy (type) (280) showed that monozygotic twins had a much higher concordance for leprosy as well as leprosy type than dizygotic ones. These results have been interpreted as indicating that genetic factors determine in part but not entirely the individuals' predisposition to leprosy (type). Not inconsistent with this view were the results from complex analyses suggesting a multi-factorial model for genetic susceptibility to leprosy (281, 282).

The presence of polymorphic MHC Ir genes in experimental animals, and the rapidly increasing number of HLA and disease associations provided a major impetus to the search for HLA encoded genetic factors which were related with susceptibility or resistance to leprosy. Basically, two approaches were used: (i) population studies, which concentrated on associations between particular HLA specificities and leprosy and (ii) family studies, in which the segregation of parental HLA-haplotypes to children were studied.

1. Population studies of HLA class I and class II specificities in leprosy.

The early population studies compared the distributions of the HLA-A, -B and -C antigens between patients of different leprosy types and healthy controls (283-301). Most of these studies observed an increase or decrease of a certain HLA specificity in patients compared to controls. However, most of these associations were weak and confined to the population tested only and in several cases were not reproducible. This lack of convincing associations between HLA class I alleles and leprosy may imply that the class I specificities are not the right markers for HLA encoded Ir/Is genes.

More convincing and consistent data were found when the HLA class II specificities were studied. A number of studies on sporadic TT leprosy cases demonstrated an increased frequency of DR2 (251,302-306) as well as DQw1 (251,303-306). A negative study with respect to sporadic TT leprosy was reported in India (307) where in the same area DR2 was associated with familiar TT leprosy (308, 309). One report showed a decreased frequency of DR4 and MT3 (DRw53) (305) whereas DR3 was increased in Surinam TT patients (189). In a Chinese study, A9-DR2, A11-DR5 and Bw60-DR3 haplotypes occurred more frequently among TT leprosy patients (310). With regard to (BL-)LL leprosy, several studies reported associations of DR2 and DQw1 (251,303,304,310,311) or of DQw1 alone (see table 1) with this type

Table 1

Relative risks, chi-squares and p-values for HLA-DR and -DQ specificities in Venezuelan lepromatous leprosy patients and healthy controls.

Antigen	Patients +	Patients −	Controls +	Controls −	RR	χ^2	p-value
HLA-DR1	9	23	5	27	2.021	1.439	0.288
-DR2	11	21	6	26	2.180	1.969	0.157
-DR3	4	28	3	29	1.330	0.157	0.693
-DR4	13	19	13	19	1.000	0.000	1.000
-DR5	8	24	9	23	0.858	0.079	0.774
-DRw6	5	27	6	26	0.815	0.108	0.740
-DR7	9	23	10	22	0.866	0.074	0.781
-DRw8	2	30	6	26	0.334	2.202	0.134
-DRw52	17	15	22	10	0.526	1.626	0.199
-DRw53	19	13	21	11	0.772	0.265	0.612
-DQw1	21	11	13	19	2.700	3.944	0.044
-DQw2	12	20	13	19	0.880	0.065	0.793
-DQw3	21	11	19	13	1.294	0.265	0.612

Note: DRw9 and w10 negative in patients and controls.
Data taken from ref. 320.

of leprosy. Interestingly, DQw1 was associated with lepromin negative familiar leprosy cases (312). One study observed a (not significant) increased frequency of DR5 in BL-LL leprosy in northern Thailand (306) whereas another one reported a decrease of DRw9 and MT3 (DRw53) in Japanese LL patients (304). Of particular interest may be the frequency of DR3 in BL-LL leprosy in Surinam which was decreased in contrast to the situation in TT leprosy as mentioned (189).

Thus, the associations between HLA class II alleles and TT as well as BL-LL leprosy are more consistent and convincing than those in the case of class I antigens. It therefore seems that class II products may be better markers for the postulated HLA Ir/Is genes, and these genes thus might map closer to the class II than to the class I region.

Besides the association studies of leprosy types and HLA, a few studies analyzed the influence of HLA specificities on skin test responses against *M. leprae* and related mycobacteria. One as mentioned described an association of DQw1 with lepromin negative leprosy in familiar cases (312); another one reported the absence of DR3 among healthy British individuals who were nonresponders against all mycobacterial antigens tested (183). DR3 was increased, albeit not significantly, in those individuals that responded to all mycobacteria, designated as common mycobacterial antigen reactors. Interestingly, an association of DR3 with high skin test responsiveness against *M. leprae* was observed in Ethiopian borderline tuberculoid leprosy patients with a history of reversal reactions (figure 4). Since DR3 was not associated with borderline tuberculoid leprosy and/or reversal reactions per se, the observed DR3 associated high responsiveness to *M. leprae* does not seem to be an etiological factor in the development of borderline tuberculoid leprosy and/or reversal reactions. Another study on HLA and skin test responsiveness is described in this thesis (chapter 7). Thus, in conclusion, HLA class II encoded genes and products may be involved in determining the type of leprosy which develops in patients as well as the type of skin test response to intradermally injected *M. leprae* (and related mycobacterial) antigens, both in leprosy patients and in healthy controls.

2. Segregation of HLA haplotypes in multicase leprosy families.

In contrast to population studies which rely on the linkage disequilibrium of the studied marker with a particular gene locus, family studies address the segregation of complete haplotypes and thus may reveal genetic control even in the absence of a detectable association at the population level, e.g. when no markers can be found in a sufficiently strong linkage disequilibrium with the gene locus of interest.

A number of family studies have been performed with respect to tuberculoid leprosy. In the first study carried out in Surinam, a significant non-random

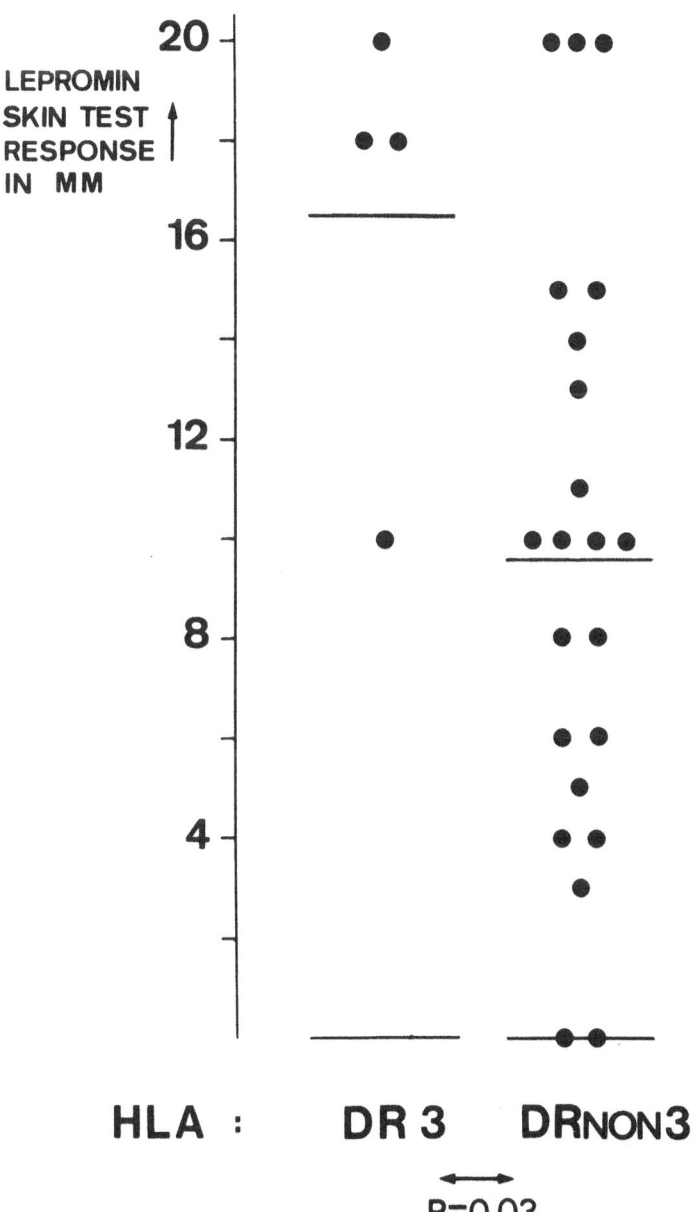

Fig. 4
Differences in the distribution of the lepromin skin test results between HLA-DR3 positive and HLA-DR3 negative (non 3) borderline tuberculoid leprosy patients with a history of reversal reactions. The resulting p-value was derived from the Mann Whitney rank sum test. No significant differences were observed for the other HLA-DR specificities. The mean skin test diameters are indicated. The data are taken from ref. 321.

segregation of HLA haplotypes was observed in multicase tuberculoid leprosy families, with an excess of shared haplotypes among affected children (313). Similar observations were made in three other studies in India (308,309,314). The results were compatible with recessive HLA linked factors predisposing to TT leprosy. Another analysis on these and other data, namely a classical linkage analysis by the method of lod scoring, supported this notion (315). Also more recent haplotype segregation studies were consistent with this recessive model (311,316).

Not until recently such family studies addressed multicase BL-LL families as well. Whereas initially HLA linked factors were thought to predispose to TT leprosy only, these studies clearly provided evidence in favour of HLA linked control of predisposition to lepromatous leprosy (311,312,316,317). An analysis of the pooled data of several of the mentioned family studies indicated that the non-random HLA haplotype segregation in multicase TT or BL-LL families was confined to affected children only, but was perfectly random in their healthy siblings. If HLA linked genes would have conferred susceptibility to leprosy per se, one would have expected a preferential – and thus non-random – segregation of parental haplotypes lacking such HLA linked susceptibility genes to healthy sibs. The mentioned random segregation in healthy sibs however thus suggests that HLA linked genes do not confer susceptibility to leprosy per se but rather determine the type of leprosy that develops upon infection in – genetically or otherwise – susceptible individuals (318).

Finally, in some of the mentioned family studies a preferential inheritance of HLA haplotypes carrying a certain class II specificity was observed. DR2 haplotypes segregated preferentially to TT affected children in the Indian studies (308,309) although as mentioned there was no excess of DR2 in TT patients at the population level (307). In the Venezuelan families, a significant deficit of DR3 haplotypes was observed among BL-LL children, whereas DR3-haplotypes tended to be inherited more often although not significant by TT cases (316), remarkably parallelling the findings in the mentioned Surinam population study. On the other hand, DQw1 positive haplotypes segregated preferentially to BL-LL affected children. It is interesting that such a preferential DQw1 haplotype segregation to BL-LL children has also been noted in a Chinese population (see table 2). As mentioned, the same observation was made for lepromin negative leprosy affected children in another study (312).

Thus, in summary, family studies have indicated that HLA linked genes presumably do not control susceptibility to leprosy per se but control – in part – the type of leprosy that may develop upon infection, at least for TT and BL-LL leprosy. Population studies have provided HLA class II markers for leprosy types. Skin test studies have suggested a role for HLA class II genes in controlling the type of immune response to *M. leprae* and closely related mycobacteria. Thus, the HLA class II region may well encode Ir and/

41

or Is genes for *M. leprae* antigens, that presumably determine the type of T cell mediated immune reactivity against the bacillus. This supposition, the availability of defined *M. leprae* antigens and the possibility of isolating the mentioned *M. leprae* reactive T cells from leprosy patients have provided the basis for the studies discussed in this thesis.

Table 2

Preferential inheritance of DQw1 haplotypes by lepromatous and of DQnon1 haplotypes by tuberculoid leprosy affected children in Chinese multicase leprosy families[1].

Leprosy status children	DQw1 inherited	DQw1 not inherited	p-value[2]
BT/TT leprosy	2	8	} 0.003
BL/LL leprosy	9	1	
healthy[3]	10	11	} 0.03

Notes.
1. R.R.P. de Vries *et al.*, unpublished observations. Preference for DQw1 or DQnon1 haplotype segregation was studied in case of DQw1/non1 heterozygous parents. The families studied have been described in ref. 317.
2. p-value derived from χ^2 test.
3. Only healthy children older than the youngest affected sib in that family were included in the analysis.

References

1. Dausset, J. 1954. Vox Sang. 6:190-198.
2. Miescher, P. and Fauconnet, M. 1954. Schweiz. Med. Wschr. 84: 597-599.
3. Van Rood, J.J., Eernisse, J.G. and Van Leeuwen, A. 1958. Nature 181: 1735-1736.
4. Payne, R. and Rolfs, M.R. 1958. J. Clin. Invest. 37: 1756-1763.
5. Van Rood, J.J. and Van Leeuwen, A. 1963. J. Clin. Invest. 42: 1382-1390.
6. Payne, R., Tripp, M., Weigle, J., Bodmer, W.F. and Bodmer J. 1964. Cold Spring Harb. Symp. Quant. Biol., vol. 29, pp 285-295.
7. Ceppellini, R., Curtoni, E.S. Mattiuz, P.L. Miggiano, V., Scudeler, G. and Serra, A. 1967. In: *Histocompatibility Testing 1967*. (Eds. Curtoni, E.S., Mattiuz, P.C. and Tosi, R.J.) Munksgaard, Copenhagen, pp. 147-187.
8. Kissmeyer-Nielsen, F., Svejgaard, A., Ahrons, S. and Staub Nielsen, L. 1969. Nature 224: 75-76.
9. Van Rood, J.J., Van Leeuwen, A. and Bruning, J.W. 1967. J. Clin. Path. 20 (suppl.): 504-512.
10. Singal, D.P., Mickey, M.R. and Terasaki, P.I. 1969. Transplantation 7: 246-258.
11. Götze, D. 1977. *The major histocompatibility system in man and animals*. Springer Verlag, Berlin.
12. Van Someren, H., Westerveld, A., Hagemeyer, A., Mees, J.R., Meera Khan, P. and Zaalberg, O.B. 1974. Proc. Natl. Acad. Sci. USA 71: 962-965.
13. De Vries, R.R.P. and Van Rood, J.J. 1985. Progr. Allergy 36: 1-9.
14. Möller, G. 1985. Immunol. Rev., vol. 87.
15. White, P.C. Grossberger, D., Onufer, B.J., Chaplin, D.D., New, M.I., Dupont, B. and Strominger, J.L. 1985. Proc. Natl. Acad. Sci. USA 82: 1089-1093.
16. Srivastava, R., Duceman, B.W., Biro, P.A., Sood, A.K. and Weissman, S.M. 1985. Immunol. Rev. 84: 93-121.
17. Goodfellow, P.N., Jones, E.A., Van Heijningen, V., Solomon, E., Bobrow, M., Migiano, V. and Bodmer, W.F. 1975. Nature 254: 267-269.
18. Orr, H.T., Lopez de Castro, J.A., Parham, P., Ploegh, H.L. and Strominger, J.L., 1979. Proc. Natl. Acad. Sci. USA 76: 4395-4399.
19. Kaufman, J.F., Auffray, C., Korman, A.J., Shackelford, D.A. and Strominger, J.L. 1984. Cell 36: 1-13.
20. Korman, A.J., Boss, J.M, Spies, T., Sorrentino, R., Okada, K. and Strominger, J.L. 1985. Immunol. Rev. 85: 45-86.
21. Trowsdale, J., Young, J.A.T., Kelly, A.P., Austin, P.J., Carson, S., Meunier, H., So, A., Erlich, H.A., Spielman, R.S., Bodmer, J. and Bodmer, W.F. 1985. Immunol. Rev. 85: 5-43.
22. Figueroa, F. and Klein, J. 1986. Immunol. Today 7: 78-81.
23. Trowsdale, J., Kelly, A., Lee, J., Carson, S., Austin, P. and Bodmer, W.F. 1984. Cell 38: 241-249.
24. Okada, K., Boss, J., Prentice, H., Spies, T., Mengler, R., Auffray, C., Lillie, J., Grossberger, D. and Strominger, J.L. 1985. Proc. Natl. Acad. Sci. USA 82: 3410-3414.
25. Böhme, J., Owerbach, D., Devano, M., Lernmark, A., Peterson, P.A. and Rask, L. 1983. Nature 301: 82-84.
26. Segall, M., Cairns, J.S., Dahl, C.A., Curtsinger, J.M., Freeman, S., Nelson, P.J., Cohen, O., Wu, S., Nicklas, J.N., Noreen, H.J., Linner, K.M., Saunders, T.L., Choong, S.A., Ohta, N., Reinsmoen, N.L., Alter, B.J. and Bach, F.H. 1985. Immunol. Rev. 85: 129-148.
27. Tonnelle, C., DeMars, R. and Long, E.O. 1985. Embo J. 4: 2839-2847.
28. Trowsdale, J. and Kelly, A. 1985. Embo J. 4: 2231-2237.
29. Hardy, D., Bell, J.I., Long, E., Lindsten, T. and McDevitt, H.O. 1986. Abstract 6th International Congress of Immunology, Toronto 1986, p. 140.
30. Böhme, J., Andersson, M., Andersson, G., Möller, E., Peterson, P.A. and Rask, L. 1985. J. Immunol. 135: 2149-2155.

31. Bontrop, R.E., Schreuder, G.M.Th., Elferink, D.G., Mikulski, M.M.A., Geerse, R. and Giphart, M.J. 1986. J. Immunol. 137: 211-216.
32. Slierendrecht, B. Personal communication.
33. Germain, R.N. and Quill, H. 1986. Nature 320: 72-75.
34. Charron, D.J., Lotteau, V. and Turmel, P. 1984. Nature 312: 157-160.
35. Germain, R.N., Bentley, D.M. and Quill, H. 1985. Cell 43: 233-242.
36. Kvist, S., Wiman, K., Claesson, L., Peterson, P.A. and Dobberstein, B. 1982. Cell 29: 61-69.
37. Robinson, J., Sieff, C., Delia, D., Edwards, P. and Greaves, M. 1981. Nature 289: 68-71.
38. Falkenburg, J.H.F., Fibbe, W.E., Goselink, H.M., Van Rood, J.J. and Jansen, J. 1985. J. Exp. Med. 162: 1359-1369.
39. Groenewegen, G., Buurman, W.A. and Van der Linden, C.J. 1985. Nature 316: 361-363.
40. Cerf-Bensussan, N., Quaroni, A., Kurnick, J., and Bahn, A. 1984. J. Immunol. 132: 2244-2252.
41. Daynes, R.A., Emam, M., Krueger, G.G. and Roberts, L.K. 1983. J. Immunol. 130: 1536-1539.
42. Pujol-Borrell, R., Hanafusa, T., Chiovato, L. and Bottazzo, G.F. 1983. Nature 304: 71-73.
43. Massa, P.T., Dörries, R. and Ter Meulen, V. 1986. Nature 320: 543-546.
44. Pober, J.S., Collins, T., Gimbrone, J.R., Cotran, R.S., Gitlin, J.D., Fiers, W., Clayberger, C., Krensky, A.M., Burakoff, S.J. and Reiss, C.S. 1983. Nature 305: 726-729.
45. Basham, T. and Merigan, T. 1983. J. Immunol. 130: 1492-1494.
46. Snyder, D., Beller, D. and Unanue, E. 1982. Nature 299: 163-165.
47. Schuurman, R.K.B., Van Rood, J.J., Vossen, J.M., Schellekens, P.T.A., Feltkamp-Vroom, T.M., Doyer, E., Gmelig-Meyling, F. and Visser, H.K.A. 1979. Clin. Immunol. Immunopathol. 14: 418-434.
48. De Préval, C., Lisowska-Grospierre, B., Loche, M., Griscelli, C. and Mach, B. 1985. Nature 318: 291-293.
49. Klein, J. and Figueroa, F. 1986. Immunol. Today 7: 41-44.
50. Hood, L., Steinmetz, M. and Malissen, B. 1983. Ann. Rev. Immunol. 1: 529-568.
51. Weiss, E., Golden, L., Fahrner, K., Mellor, A., Devlin, J., Bullman, H., Tiddens, H., Bud, H. and Flavell, R. 1984. Nature 310: 650-655.
52. Mellor, A. 1986. Immunol. Today 7: 19-24.
53. Gazit, E., Terhorst, C. and Yunis, E.J. 1980. Nature 284: 275-277.
54. Van Leeuwen, A., Festenstein, H. and Van Rood, J.J. 1980. J. Exp. Med. 152: 235S-242S.
55. Van Leeuwen, A., Festenstein, H. and Van Rood, J.J. 1982. Human Immunol. 4: 109-121.
56. Zinkernagel, R.M. and Doherty, P.C. 1974. Nature 248: 701-702.
57. Rosenthal, A.S. and Shevach, E.M. 1973. J. Exp. Med. 138: 1194-1212.
58. Zinkernagel, R.M. and Doherty, P.C. 1979. Adv. Immunol. 27: 51-177.
59. Kaufmann, S.H.E. and Hahn, H. 1982. J. Exp. Med. 140: 648-659.
60. Thorsby, E. 1984. Human Immunol. 9: 1-7.
61. Bloom, B.R. and Godal, T. 1983. Rev. Infect. Dis. 5: 765-780.
62. Schwartz, R.H. 1985. Ann. Rev. Immunol. 3: 237-261.
63. Schwartz, R.H. 1986. Adv. Immunol. 38: 31-202.
64. Unanue, E.R. 1984. Ann. Rev. Immunol. 2: 395-428.
65. Ziegler, H.K. and Unanue, E.R. 1982. Proc. Natl. Acad. Sci. USA. 79: 175-178.
66. Grey, H.M. and Chestnut, R.S. 1985. Immunol. Today 6: 101-106.
67. Shimonkewitz, R., Kappler, J.W., Marrack, P. and Grey, H.M. 1983. J. Exp. Med. 158: 303-316.
68. Streicher, H.Z., Berkower, I.J., Busch, M., Gurd, F.R.N. and Berzofsky, J.A. 1984. Proc. Natl. Acad. Sci. USA 81: 6831-6835.
69. Heber-Katz, E., Hollosi, M., Dietzschold, B., Hudecz, F. and Fasman, G.D. 1985. J. Immunol. 135: 1385-1390.

70. Schwartz, R.H., Fox, B.S., Fraga, E., Chen, C. and Singh, B. 1985. J. Immunol. 135: 2598-2608.
71. Walden, P., Nagy, Z.A. and Klein, J. 1985. Nature 315: 327-329.
72. Allen, P.M. and Unanue, E.R. 1984. J. Immunol. 132: 1077-1079.
73. Shimonkewitz, R., Colon, S., Kappler, J.W., Marrack, P. and Grey, H.M. 1984. J. Immunol. 133: 2067-2074.
74. Allen, P.M., Strydom, D.J. and Unanue, E.R. 1984. Proc. Natl. Acad. Sci. USA 81: 2489-2493.
75. Berkower, I., Buckenmeyer, G.K. and Berzofsky, J.A. 1986. J. Immunol. 136: 2498-2503.
76. DeLisi, C. and Berzofsky, J.A. 1985. Proc. Natl. Acad. Sci. USA 82: 7048-7052.
77. Goodman, J.W. and Sercarz, E.E. 1983. Ann. Rev. Immunol. 1: 465-498.
78. Benjamin, D.C., Berzofsky, J.A. East, I.J., Gurd, F.R.N., Hannum, C., Leach, S.J., Margoliash, E., Michael, J.G., Miller, A., Prager, E.M., Reichlin, M., Sercarz, E.E., Smith-Gill, S.J., Todd, P.E. and Wilson, A.C. 1984. Ann. Rev. Immunol. 2: 67-101.
79. Adorini, L., Harvey, M.A., Miller, A. and Sercarz, E.E. 1979. J. Exp. Med. 150: 293-306.
80. Krzych, K., Fowler, A.V. and Sercarz, E.E. 1985. J. Exp. Med. 162: 311-323.
81. Hashim, G.A. 1978. Immunol. Rev. 39: 60-107.
82. Beller, D.I. 1984. Eur. J. Immunol. 14: 138-143.
83. Janeway, C.A., Bottomly, K., Babich, J., Conrad, P., Conzen, S., Jones, B., Kaye, J., Katz, M., McVay, L., Murphy, D.B. and Tite, J. 1984. Immunol. Today 5: 99-105.
84. Bontrop, R.E., Ottenhoff, T.H.M., Van Miltenburg, R., Elferink, D.G., De Vries, R.R.P. and Giphart, M.J. 1985. Eur. J. Immunol. 16: 133-138.
85. Fathman, C.G., Kimoto, M., Melvold, R., and David, C.S. 1981. Proc. Natl. Acad. Sci. USA 78: 1853-1857.
86. Glimcher, L.H., Sharrow, S.O. and Paul, W.E. 1983. J. Exp. Med. 158: 1573-1588.
87. Brown, M.A., Glimcher, L.A., Nielsen, E.A., Paul, W.E. and Germain, R.N. 1986. Science 231: 255-258.
88. Austin, P., Trowsdale, J., Rudd, C., Bodmer, W., Feldmann, M. and Lamb, J. 1985. Nature 313: 61-64.
89. Watts, T.H., Brian, A.A., Kappler, J.W., Marrack, P. and McConnell, H.M. 1984. Proc. Natl. Acad. Sci. USA 81: 7564-7568.
90. Ashwell, J.D., De Franco, A.L., Paul, W.E. and Schwartz, R.H. 1984. J. Exp. Med. 159: 881-905.
91. Chestnut, R.W., Colon, S.M. and Grey, H.M. 1982. J. Immunol. 128: 1764-1768.
92. Elferink, B.G., Ottenhoff, T.H.M. and De Vries, R.R.P. 1985. Scand. J. Immunol. 22: 585-589.
93. Hirschberg, H., Braathen, L.R. and Thorsby, E. 1982. Immunol. Rev. 66: 57-77.
94. Umetsu, D.T., Katzen, D., Jabara, H.H. and Geha, R.S. 1986. J. Immunol. 136: 440-445
95. Londei, M., Lamb, J.R., Bottazzo, G.F. and Feldmann, M. 1984. Nature 312: 639-641.
96. Scala, G., Allavena, P., Ortaldo, J.R., Herberman, R.B. and Oppenheim, J.J. 1985. J. Immunol. 134: 3049-3055.
97. Triebel, F., De Rocquefeuil, S., Blanc, C., Charron, D.J. and Debré, P. 1986. Human Immunol. 15: 302-315.
98. Hanafusa, T., Pujol-Borrell, R., Chiovatto, L., Russell, R.C.G., Doniach, D. and Bottazzo, G.F. 1983. Lancet ii: 1111-1114.
99. Ballardini, G., Mirakian, R., Bianchi, F.B., Pisi, E., Doniach, D. and Bottazzo, G.F. 1984. Lancet ii: 1009-1012.
100. Inaba, K. and Steinman, R.M. 1985. Science 229: 475-479.
101. Duram, S.K., Schmidt, J.A. and Oppenheim, J.J. 1985. Ann. Rev. Immunol. 3: 263-287.
102. Malissen, B. 1986. Immunol. Today 7: 106-112.
103. Le Meur, M., Gerlinger, P., Benoist, C. and Mathis, D. 1985. Nature 316: 38-42.
104. Yamamura, K., Kikutani, H., Folsom, V., Clayton, L.K., Kimoto, M., Akira, S., Kashiwamura, S., Tonegawa, S. and Kishimoto, T. 1985. Nature 316: 67-69.

105. Lin, C., Rosenthal, A.S., Passmore, H.C. and Hansen, T.H. 1981. Proc. Natl. Acad. Sci. USA 78: 6406-6410.
106. Baxevanis, C.N., Ishii, N., Nagy, Z.A. and Klein, J. 1982. J. Exp. Med. 156: 822-833.
107. Berkower, I., Kawamura, H., Matis, L.A. and Berzofsky, J.A. 1985. J. Immunol. 135: 2628-2634.
108. Durandy, A., Fisher, A., Charron, D.J. and Griscelli, C. 1986. Human Immunol. 16: 114-125.
109. Sasazuki, T., Tsukamoto, K., Kikuchi, I., Hirayama, K., Matsushita, S. and Yasunami, M. 1986. Abstract 6th International Congress of Immunology, Toronto 1986, p. 584.
110. Paäbo, S., Kämpe, O., Severinsson, L., Andersson, M., Fernandez, C. and Peterson, P.A. 1985. Progr. Allergy 36: 114-134.
111. Claas, F.H.J. and Van Rood, J.J. 1985. Progr. Allergy 36: 135-150.
112. Werderlin, O. 1982. J. Immunol. 129: 1883-1891.
113. Rock, K.L. and Benacerraf, B. 1983. J. Exp. Med. 157: 1618-1634.
114. Rock, K.L. and Benacerraf, B. 1984. J. Exp. Med. 160: 1864-1879.
115. Rock, K.L. and Benacerraf, B. 1984. J. Exp. Med. 159: 1238-1252.
116. Heber-Katz, E., Schwartz, R.H., Matis, L.A., Hannum, C., Fairwell, T., Appella, E. and Hansburg, D. 1982. J. Exp. Med. 155: 1086-1099.
117. Heber-Katz, E., Hansburg, D. and Schwartz, R.H. 1983. J. Mol. Cell. Immunol. 1: 3-14
118. Babbitt, B.P., Allen, P.M., Matsueda, G., Haber, E. and Unanue, E.R. 1985. Nature 317: 359-361.
119. Buus, S., Freed, J.H. and Grey, H.M. 1986. Abstract 6th International Congress of Immunology, Toronto 1986, p. 147.
120. Ashwell, J.D. and Schwartz, R.H. 1986. Nature 320: 176-179.
121. Watts, T.H., Gaub, H.E. and McConnell, H.M. 1986. Nature 320: 179-181.
122. Friedman, A., Zerubavel, R., Gitler, C. and Cohen, I.R. 1983. Immunogenetics 18: 291-302.
123. Marrack, P. and Kappler, J. 1986. Adv. Immunol. 38: 1-30.
124. Meuer, S.C., Fitzgerald, K.A., Hussey, R.E., Hodgdon, J.C., Schlossmann, S.F. and Reinherz, E.L. 1983. J. Exp. Med. 157: 705-719.
125. Meuer, S.C., Hodgdon, J.C., Hussey, R.E., Protentis, J.P., Schlossmann, S.F. and Reinherz, E.L. 1983. J. Exp. Med. 158: 988-993.
126. Hedrick, S., Cohen, D., Nielsen, E. and Davis, M. 1984. Nature 308: 149-153.
127. Yanagi, Y., Yoshikai, Y., Leggett, K., Clark, S., Alexander, I. and Mak, T. 1984. Nature 308: 145-149.
128. Saito, H., Kranz, D.M., Takagaki, Y., Hayday, A.C., Eisen, H.N., and Tonegawa, S. 1984. Nature 312: 36-40.
129. Brenner, M.B., McLean, J., Dialynas, D.P., Strominger, J.L., Smith, J.A., Owen, F.L., Seidman, J.G., Ip, S., Rosen, F. and Krangel, M.S. 1986. Nature 322: 145-149.
130. Bank, I., DePinho, R.A., Brenner, M.B., Cassimeris, J., Alt, F.W. and Chess, L. 1986. Nature 322: 179-181.
131. Dembic, Z., Haas, W., Weiss, S., McCubrey, J., Kiefer, H., Von Boehmer, H. and Steinmetz, M. 1986. Nature 320: 232-238.
132. Borst, J., Coligan, J.E., Oettgen, H., Persano, S., Malni, R. and Terhorst, C. 1984. Nature 312: 455-458.
133. Oettgen, H.C., Pettey, C.L., Maloy, W.L. and Terhorst, C. 1986. Nature 320: 272-275.
134. Fink, P.J., Matis, L.A., McElligott, D.L., Bookman, M. and Hedrick, S.M. 1986. Nature 321: 219-226.
135. Ready, A.R., Jenkinson, E.J., Kingston, R. and Owen, J.J.T. 1984. Nature 310: 231-233.
136. Kast, W.M., De Waal, L.P. and Melief, C.J.M. 1984. J. Exp. Med. 160: 1752-1766.
137. Klein, J. (Ed.) 1982. *Immunology: the science of self- non self discrimination*. Wiley, New York.
138. Meuer, S.C., Hussey, R.E., Fabbi, M., Fox, D., Acuto, O., Fitzgerald, K.A. Hodgdon, J.C., Protentis, J.P., Schlossmann, S.F. and Reinherz, E.L. 1984. Cell 36: 897-906.

139. Hara, T., Man Fu, S. and Hansen, J.A. 1985. J. Exp. Med. 161: 1513-1524.
140. Milanese, C., Richardson, N.E. and Reinherz, E.L. 1986. Science 231: 1118-1122.
141. Truneh, A., Albert, F., Goldstein, P. and Schmitt-Verhulst, A. 1985. Nature 313: 318-320.
142. O'Flynn, K., Kremsky, A.M., Beverly, P.C.L., Burakoff, S.J. and Linch, D.C. 1985. Nature 313: 686-687.
143. Smith, K.A. 1984. Ann. Rev. Immunol. 2: 319-333.
144. Nathan, C.F., Murray, H.W., Wiebe, M.E. and Rubin, B.Y. 1983. J. Exp. Med. 158: 670-689.
145. Golding, H., McCluskey, J., Munitz, T.I., Germain, R.N., Margulies, D.H. and Singer, A. 1985. Nature 317: 425-427.
146. Bank, I. and Chess, L. 1985. J. Exp. Med. 162: 1294-1303.
147. Springer, T.A., Davignnon, D., Ho, M-K., Korzinger, K., Martz, E. and Sanchez-Madrid, E. 1982. Immunol. Rev. 68: 171-195.
148. Zinkernagel, R.M., Pfau, C.J., Hengartner, H. and Althage, A. 1985. Nature 316: 814-817.
149. Kast, W.M., Bronkhorst, A.M., De Waal, L.P. and Melief, C.J.M. 1986. J. Exp. Med., in press.
150. Biozzi, G., Mouton, D., Heumann, A.M., Bouthillier, Y., Stiffel, C. and Mevel, J.C. 1979. Immunology 36: 427-438.
151. Skamene, E., Gros, P., Forget, A., Kongshavn, P.A.L., StCharles, C. and Taylor, B.A. 1982. Nature 297: 506-510.
152. Skamene, E., Gros, P., Forget, A., Patel, P.J. and Nesbitt, M.N. 1984. Immunogenetics 19: 117-124.
153. Levine, B.B., Ojeda, A. and Benacerraf, B. 1963. J. Exp. Med. 118: 953-957.
154. McDevitt, H.O. and Chinitz, A. 1969. Science 163: 1207-1209.
155. Lilly, F., Boyse, E.A. and Old, L.J. 1964. Lancet ii: 1207-1209.
156. Blackwell, J., Freeman, J. and Bradley, D. 1980. Nature 283: 72-74.
157. Adu, H.O., Curtis, J. and Turk, J.L. 1983. Infect. Immun. 40: 720-725.
158. Benacerraf, B. 1981. Science 212: 1229-1238.
159. Schwartz, R.H., David, C.S., Sachs, D.H. and Paul, W.E. 1976. J. Immunol. 117: 531-540.
160. Dorf, M.E. and Benacerraf, B. 1975. Proc. Natl. Acad. Sci. USA 72: 3671-3675.
161. Gasser, D.L. 1969. J. Immunol. 103: 66-70.
162. Waters, S.J., Waksal, S.D., Norton, G.P. and Bona, C.A. 1984. J. Exp. Med. 159: 305-312.
163. Klein, J. 1984. Immunol. Rev. 81: 177-202.
164. Nagy, Z.A., Baxevanis, C.N., Ishii, N. and Klein, J. 1981. Immunol. Rev. 60: 59-83.
165. Gammon, G., Dunn, K., Shastri, N., Oki, A., Wilbur, S. and Sercarz, E.E. 1986. Nature 319: 413-415.
166. Janeway, C.A. 1983. J. Mol. Cell. Immunol. 1: 15-19.
167. Zamvil, S., Nelson, P., Trotter, J., Mitchell, D., Knobler, R., Fritz, R. and Steinman, L. 1985. Nature 317: 355-358.
168. Hsu, S.H., Chan, M.M. and Bias, W.B. 1981. Proc. Natl. Acad. Sci. USA 78: 440-444.
169. Buckley, C.E. Dorsey, F.C., Corley, R.B., Ralph, W.B., Woodbury, M.A. and Amos, D.B. 1973. Proc. Natl. Acad. Sci. USA. 70: 2157-2161.
170. Greenberg, L.J., Gray, E.D. and Yunis, E.J. 1975. J. Exp. Med. 141: 935-943.
171. Greenberg, L.J., Chopyk, R.L., Bradley, P.W. and Lalouel, J.M. 1980. Immunogenetics 11: 161-167.
172. Nishimura, Y. and Sasazuki, T. 1983. Nature 302: 67-69.
173. Lehner, T., Lamb, J.R., Welsh, K.L. and Batchelor, J.R. 1984. Nature 292: 770-772.
174. Spencer, M.J., Cherry, J.D. and Terasaki, P.I. 1976. New Engl. J. Med. 294: 13-16.
175. De Vries, R.R.P., Kreeftenberg, H.G., Loggen, H.G. and Van Rood, J.J. 1977. New Engl. J. Med. 297: 692-696.
176. Sasazuki, T., Kokuo, Y., Iwanoto, I., Tanimura, M. and Naito, S. 1978. Nature 272: 359-361.

177. Sasazuki, T., Ohta, N., Kaneoka, R. and Kojima, S. 1980. J. Exp. Med. 152: 314S-318S.
178. Marsh, D.G., Hsu, S.H., Roebber, M., Ehrlich-Kautzky, E., Freidhoff, L.R., Meyers, D.A., Pollard, M.K. and Bias, W.B. 1982. J. Exp. Med. 155: 1439-1451.
179. Whittingham, S., Mathews, J.D., Schanfield, M.S., Matthews, J.V., Tait, B.D., Morris, P.J. and Mackay, I.R. 1980. Clin. Exp. Immunol. 40: 8-15.
180. Sasazuki, T., Nishimura, Y., Muto, M. and Ohta, N. 1983. Immunol. Rev. 70: 51-75.
181. Haverkorn, M.J., Hofman, B., Masurel, N. and Van Rood, J.J. 1975. Transplant. Rev. 22: 120-124.
182. Hensen, E.J. and Elferink, B.G. 1984. Human Immunol. 10: 113-128.
183. Van Eden, W., De Vries, R.R.P., Stanford, J.L. and Rook, G.A.W. 1983. Clin. Exp. Immunol. 52: 282-292.
184. Paty, D.W., Cousin, R.K., Stiller, C.R., Boucher, D.W., Furesz, J., Warren, K.G., Marchuk, L. and Dossetor, J.B. 1977. Transpl. Proc. 9: 1845-1848.
185. Osaba, D., Dick, H.M., Voller, A., Goosen, T.J., Goosen, T., Draper, C.C. and De The, G. 1979. Immunogenetics 8: 323-338.
186. Boyer, K.M., Sumaya, C.V. and Cherry, J.D. 1980. Tissue Antigens 15: 105-111.
187. Sasazuki, T., Nishimura, Y., Muto, M. and Saito, Y. 1984. In: *Immunogenetics. Its application to clinical medicine.* (Eds. Sasazuki, T. and Tada, T.) Academic Press, Tokyo, pp. 21-37.
188. Van Eden, W., Elferink, B.G., De Vries, R.R.P., Leiker, D.L. and Van Rood, J.J. 1984. Clin. Exp. Immunol. 55: 140-148.
189. Van Eden, W., De Vries, R.R.P., D'Amaro, J., Schreuder, G.M.Th., Leiker, D.L. and Van Rood, J.J. 1982. Human Immunol. 4: 343-350.
190. Scott, H., Hirschberg, H. and Thorsby, E. 1983. Scand. J. Immunol. 18: 163-167.
191. Svejgaard, A., Platz, P. and Ryder, L.P. 1983. Immunol. Rev. 70: 193-218.
192. Singh, S.P.N., Mehra, N.K., Dingley, H.B., Pande, J.N. and Vaidya, M.C. 1983. J. Infect. Dis. 148: 676-681.
193. Singh, S.P.N., Mehra, N.K., Dingley, H.B., Pande, J.N. and Vaidya, M.C. 1984. Tissue Antigens 23: 84-86.
194. Chan, S.H., Tan, T., Kamarudin, A., Wee, G.B. and Rajan, V.S. 1979. Brit. J. Ven. Dis. 55: 207-210.
195. Tejani, A., Mahadevan, R., Dobias, B., Nangia, B. and Weiner, M. 1981. Tissue Antigens 17: 205-211.
196. Van Eden, W., Persijn, G.G., Bijkerk, H., De Vries, R.R.P., Schuurman, R.K.B. and Van Rood, J.J. 1983. J. Infect. Dis. 147: 422-426.
197. Meredith, T.A., Smith, R.E. and Duquesnoy, R.J. 1980. Amer. J. Opthalm. 89: 70-76.
198. Geczy, A.F., Alexander, K., Bashir, H.V., Edmonds, J.P., Upfold, L. and Sullivan, J. 1983. Immunol. Rev. 70: 23-50.
199. Menser, M.A., Forrest, J.M., Honeyman, M.C. and Burgess, J.A. 1974. Lancet ii: 1508-1509.
200. Piazza, A., Belvedere, M.C., Bernoco, D., Conighi, C., Contu, L., Curtoni, E.S., Mattiuz, P.L., Mayr, W., Richiardi, P., Scudeller, G. and Ceppelini, R. 1972. In: *Histocompatibility Testing 1972.* (Eds. Dausset, J. and Colombani, J). Munksgaard, Copenhagen, pp. 73-84.
201. Londei, M., Bottazzo, G.F. and Feldmann, M. 1985. Science 228: 85-89.
202. Stastny, P., Ball, E.J., Dry, P.J. and Nunez, G. 1983. Immunol. Rev. 70: 113-153.
203. Schreuder, G.M.Th., Tilanus, M.G.J., Bontrop, R.E., Bruining, G.J., Giphart, M.J., Van Rood, J.J. and De Vries, R.R.P. 1986. J. Exp. Med. in press.
204. Bell, J., Rassenti, L., Smoot, S., Smith, K., Newby, C., Hohlfeld, R., Toyka, K., McDevitt, H.O. and Steinman, L. 1986. Lancet i: 1058-1060.
205. Report of a WHO Study Group. 1985. Technical Report Series 716, WHO, Geneva.
206. Godal, T. 1978. Progr. Allergy 25: 211-242.
207. Ridley, D.S. and Jopling, W.H. 1966. Int. J. Leprosy 34: 225-273.
208. Van Voorhis, W.C., Kaplan, G., Sarno, E.N., Horwitz, M,A., Steinman, R.M., Levis, W.R., Nogueira, N., Hair, L.S., Gattass, C.R., Arrick, B.A. and Cohn, Z.A. 1982. New. Engl. J. Med. 307: 1593-1597.

209. Narayanan, R.B., Bhutani, L.K., Sharma, A.K. and Nath, I. 1983. Clin. Exp. Immunol. 51: 421-429.
210. Modlin, R.L., Hofman, F.M., Meyer, P.R., Sharma, O.P., Taylor, C.R. and Rea, T.H. 1983. Clin. Exp. Immunol. 51: 430-438.
211. Modlin, R.L., Hofman, F.M., Horwitz, D.A., Husmann, L.A., Gillis, S., Taylor, C.R. and Rea, T.H. 1985. J. Immunol. 132: 3085-3090.
212. Kaplan, G., Van Voorhis, W.C., Sarno, E.N., Nogueira, N. and Cohn, Z.A. 1983. J. Exp. Med. 158: 1145-1159.
213. Bloom, B.R. and Mehra, V. 1984. Immunol. Rev. 80: 5-28.
214. Bjune, G. 1983. Lepr. Rev. (special issue): 61S-67S.
215. Sansonetti, P. and Lagrange, P.H. 1981. Rev. Infect. Dis. 3: 422-469.
216. Bjune, G., Barnetson, R.St.C., Ridley, D.S. and Kronvall, G. 1976. Clin. Exp. Immunol. 25: 85-94.
217. Gaugas, J.M., Rees, R.J.W., Weddell, A.G.M. and Palmer, E. 1971. Int. J. Lepr. 39: 388-395.
218. Wisniewski, H.M. and Bloom, B.R. 1975. J. Exp. Med. 141: 346-359.
219. Crawford, C.L., Evans, D.H.L. and Evans, E.M. 1974. Nature 251: 223-225.
220. Crawford, C.L., Hardwicke, P.M.D., Evans, D.H.L. and Evans, E.M. 1977. Nature 265: 457-459.
221. Mshana, R.N., Humber, D.P., Harboe, M. and Belehu, A. 1983. Clin. Exp. Immunol. 52: 441-448.
222. Bjune, G., Closs, O. and Barnetson, R.St.C. 1983. Clin. Exp. Immunol. 54: 89-297.
223. Hansen, G.A 1874. Norsk Magazin for Laegevidenskaben 4: 1-88.
224. Prasad, H.K., Singh, H. and Nath, I. 1982. Clin. Exp. Immunol. 49: 517-522.
225. Shepard, C.C. 1960. J. Exp. Med. 112: 445-454.
226. Kirchheimer, W.F. and Storrs, E.E. 1971. Int. J. Lepr. 39: 693-702.
227. Martin, L.N., Gormus, B.J., Wolf, R.H., Baskin, G.B., Gerome, P.J., Meyers, W.M., Walsh, G.P., Brown, H.L., Binford, C.H., Schalel, C.J. and Hadfield, T.L. 1983. Int. J. Lepr. 51: 665-666.
228. Young, R.A., Mehra, V., Sweetser, D., Buchanan, T.M., Clark-Curtis, J., Davis, R.W. and Bloom, B.R. 1985. Nature 316: 450-452.
229. Stewart-Tull, D.E.S. 1983. In: *The Biology of the Mycobacteria*. (Eds. Ratledge, C. and Stanford, J.L.) Academic Press, London, pp. 213-308.
230. Engers, H.D., Abe, M., Bloom, B.R., Mehra, V., Britton, W., Buchanan, T.M., Khanolkar, S.K., Young, D.B., Closs, O., Gillis, T., Harboe, M., Ivanyi, J., Kolk, A.H.J. and Shepard, C.C. 1985. Infect. Immun. 48: 603-605.
231. Young, D.B. and Buchanan, T.M. 1983. Science 221: 1057-1059.
232. Closs, O., Reitan, L.J., Negassi, K., Harboe, M. and Belehu, A. 1982. Scand. J. Immunol. 16: 103-115.
233. Shepard, C.C., Walker, L.L. and Van Landingham, R. 1978. Infect. Immun. 22: 87-93
234 Patel, P.J. and Lefford, M.J. 1978. Infect. Immun. 19: 87-93.
235. Mehra, V. and Bloom, B.R. 1979. Infect. Immun. 23: 787-794.
236. Lowe, C., Brett, S.J. and Rees, R.J.W. 1985. Clin. Exp. Immunol. 61: 336-342.
237. Orme, I.M. and Collins, F.M. 1986. J. Exp. Med. 163: 203-208.
238. Mustafa, A.S., Gill, H.K., Nerland, A., Britton, W.J., Mehra, V., Bloom, B.R., Young, R.A. and Godal, T. 1986. Nature 319: 63-66.
239. Noordeen, S.K. 1985. Lepr. Rev. 56: 1-3.
240. Van Eden, W., Holoshitz, J., Nevo, Z., Frenkel, A., Klajman, A. and Cohen, I.R. 1985. Proc. Natl. Acad. Sci. USA. 82: 5117-5120.
241. Thorns, C.J. and Morris, J.A. 1985. Clin. Exp. Immunol. 61: 323-328.
242. Stoner, G.L. 1979. Lancet ii: 994-996.
243. Waldorf, D., Sheagren, J.N., Trautman, J.R. and Block, J.B. 1966. Lancet ii: 773-776.
244. Bullock, W.E. 1968. New Engl. J. Med. 278: 298-304.

245. Reitan, L.J., Closs, O. and Belehu, A. 1982. Int. J. Lepr. 50: 455-467.
246. Smelt, A.H.M., Rees, R.J.W. and Liew, F.Y. 1981. Clin. Exp. Immunol. 44: 507-511.
247. Hirschberg, H. 1978. Clin. Exp. Immunol. 34: 46-51.
248. Nath, I., Van Rood, J.J., Mehra, N.K. and Vaidya, M.C. 1980. Clin. Exp. Immunol. 42: 203-210.
249. Sathish, M., Bhutani, L.K., Sharma, A.K. and Nath, I. 1983. Infect. Immun. 42: 890-899.
250. Stoner, G.L., Mshana, R.N., Touw, J. and Belehu, A. 1982. Scand. J. Immunol. 15: 33-48.
251. Kikuchi, I., Ozawa, T. and Sasazuki., T. 1984. In: *Histocompatibility Testing 1984* (Eds. Albert, E.D., Baur, M.P. and Mayr, W.R.) Springer Verlag, Heidelberg, p. 662.
252. Godal, T., Myrvang, B., Froland, S.S., Shao, J. and Melaku, G. 1972. Scand. J. Immunol. 1: 311-321.
253. Haregewoin, A., Mustafa, A.S., Helle, I., Waters, M.F.R., Leiker, D.L. and Godal, T. 1984. Immunol. Rev. 80: 77-86.
254. Ottenhoff, T.H.M., Elferink, B.G. and De Vries, R.R.P. 1984. Int. J. Lepr. 52: 419-422.
255. Nogueira, N., Kaplan, G., Levy, E., Sarno, E.N., Kushner, P., Granelli-Piperno, A., Vieira, L., Colomer Gould, V., Levis, W., Steinmann, R., Yip, Y.K. and Cohn, Z.A. 1983. J. Exp. Med. 158: 2165-2170.
256. Nath, I., Sathish, M., Jayaraman, T., Bhutani, L.K. and Sharma, A.K. 1984. Clin. Exp. Immunol. 58: 522-530.
257. Kaplan, G., Weinstein, D.E., Steinman, R.M., Levis, W.R., Elvers, U., Patarroyo, M.E. and Cohn, Z.A. 1985. J. Exp. Med. 162: 917-929.
258. Mohagheghpour, N., Gelber, R.H., Larrick, J.W., Sasaki, D.T., Brennan, P.J. and Engleman, E.G. 1985. J. Immunol. 135: 1443-1449.
259. Shankar, P., Wallach, D. and Bach, M-A. 1986. Int. J. Lepr. 53: 649-652.
260. Barnass, S., Mace, J., Steele, J., Torres, P., Gervasoni, B., Ravioli, R., Terencio, J., Rook, G.A.W. and Waters, M.F.R. 1986. Clin. Exp. Immunol. 64: 41-49.
261. Touw, J., Stoner, G.L. and Belehu, A. 1980. Clin. Exp. Immunol. 41: 397-405.
262. Bjune, G. 1979. Clin. Exp. Immunol. 36: 479-487.
263. Nath, I. and Singh, R. 1980. Clin. Exp. Immunol. 41: 406-414.
264. Stoner, G.L., Touw, J., Atlaw, T. and Belehu, A. 1981. Lancet ii: 1372-1377.
265. Mehra, V., Mason, L.H., Fields, J.P. and Bloom, B.R. 1979. J. Immunol. 123: 1813-1817.
266. Mehra, V., Mason, L.H., Rothman, W., Reinherz, E., Schlossman, S.F. and Bloom, B.R. 1980. J. Immunol. 125: 1183-1188.
267. Mehra, V., Convit, J., Rubinstein, A. and Bloom, B.R. 1982. J. Immunol. 129: 1946-1951.
268. Mehra, V., Brennan, P.J., Rada, E., Convit, J. and Bloom, B.R. 1984. Nature 308: 194-196.
269. Prasad, II.K. and Nath, I. 1986. Abstract 6th International Congress of Immunology, Toronto 1986, p. 615.
270. Nath, I., Jayaraman, T., Sathish, M., Bhutani, L.K. and Sharma, A.K. 1984. Clin. Exp. Immunol. 58: 531-538.
271. Bach, M-A., Chatenoud, L., Wallach, D., Tuy, F.P.D. and Cottenot, F. 1981. Clin. Exp. Immunol. 44: 491-500.
272. Salgame, P.R., Mahadevan, P.R. and Antia, N.H. 1983. Infect. Immun. 40: 1119-1126.
273. Birdi, T.J., Mistry, N.F., Mahadevan, P.R. and Antia, N.H. 1983. Infect. Immun. 41: 121-127.
274. Mistry, N.F., Birdi, T.J., Mahadevan, P.R. and Antia, N.H. 1985. Scand. J. Immunol. 22: 415-423.
275. Morton, A., Nye, P., Rook, G.A.W., Samuel, N. and Stanford, J.L. 1984. Lepr. Rev. 55: 273-281.
276. Fine, P.E.M. 1981. Int. J. Lepr. 49: 437-454.
277. Aycock, W.L. and McKinley, E.B. 1938. Int. J. Lepr. 6: 169-184.
278. Spickett, S.G. 1962. Lepr. Rev. 33: 76-93, 173-181.
279. Beiguelman, B. 1972. Acta Genet. Med. Gamellol. 21: 21-52.

280. Chakravartti, M.R. and Vogel, F.A. 1973. Top. Hum. Genet. 1: 1-123.
281. Smith, D.G. 1979. Hum. Genet. 50: 163-177.
282. Serjeantson, S.W., Wilson, S.R. and Keats, B.J. 1979. Ann. Hum. Biol. 6: 375-393.
283. Thorsby, E., Godal, T. and Myrvang, B. 1973. Tissue Antigens 3: 373-377.
284. Escobar-Guttièrrez, A., Gorodezky, C. and Salazar-Mallén, M. 1973. Vox Sang. 25: 151-155.
285. Kreisler, M., Arnaiz, A., Perez, B., Fernandez Cruz, E. and Bootello, A. 1974. Tissue Antigens 4: 197-201.
286. Reis, A.P., Maia, F., Reis, V.F., Andrade, I.M. and Campos, A.A.S. 1974. Lancet ii: 1384.
287. Smith, G.S., Walford, R.L., Shepard, C.C., Payne, R. and Prochazka, G.J. 1975. Vox Sang. 28: 42-49.
288. Dasgupta, A., Mehra, N.K., Ghei, S.K. and Vaidya, M.C. 1975. Tissue Antigens 5: 85-87.
289. Rea, T.H., Levan, N.E. and Terasaki, P.I. 1976. J. Infect. Dis. 134: 615-618.
290. Mehra, N.K., Dasgupta, A., Ghei, S.K., Nilikanta Rao, M.S. and Vaidya, M.C. 1976. Microbios. Letters 3: 79-83.
291. Nakajima, S., Kobayashi, S., Nohara, M. and Sato, S. 1977. Int. J. Lepr. 45: 273-277.
292. Youngchaiyud, U., Chandanayingyong, D. and Vibhatavanija, T. 1977. Vox Sang. 32: 342-345.
293. Takata, H., Sada, M., Ozawa, S. and Sekiguchi, S. 1978. Tissue Antigens 11: 61-64.
294. Greiner, J., Schleiermacher, E., Smith, T., Lenhard, V. and Vogel, F. 1978. Hum. Genet. 42: 201-203.
295. Massoud, A., Nikbin, B., Nazari, G.R., Syadat, N.A. and Ala, F. 1978. Int. J. Lepr. 46: 149-153.
296. Chiewsilp, P., Ashkambhira, S., Chirachariyavey, T., Bhamarapravati and Entwistle, C. 1979. Tissue Antigens 13: 186-188.
297. Chan, S.H., Oon, B.B., Kamarudin, A. and Wee, G.B. 1979. Tissue Antigens 13: 73-74.
298. Mohagheghpour, N., Tabatabai, H., Mohammed, K., Ramanujam, K., and Modabber, F.Z. 1979. Int. J. Lepr. 47: 597-600.
299. Bale, U.M., Mehta, M.M., Contractor, N.M., Bhatia, H.M. and Koticha, K.K. 1982. Tissue Antigens 20: 141-143.
300. Chang, Z.N., Tsai, L.C. and Han, S.H. 1980. Chung-hua-min-kuo-wei-sheng-wu-chi-mien-I-hsueh-tsa-chih 13: 9-14.
301. Wolf, E., Fine, P.E.M., Pritchard, J., Watson, B., Bradley, D.J., Festenstein, H., Chacko, C.J.G. and Stevens, A. 1980. Tissue Antigens 15: 436-446.
302. Rea, T.H. and Terasaki, P.I. 1980. Lepr. Rev. 51: 117-123.
303. Serjeantson, S.W., Vaidya, M.C., Chan, S.H., Juji, G.T., Mehra, N.K., Naik, S. and Sasazuki, T. 1981. In: Proceedings of the second Asia and Oceania Histocompatibility Workshop Conference 1981. (Eds. Simons, M.J. and Tait, B.D.). Immunopublishing, Victoria, pp. 379-401.
304. Izumi, S., Sugiyama, K., Matsumoto, Y. and Ohkawa, S. 1982. Vox Sang. 42: 243-247.
305. Miyanaga, K., Juji, T., Maeda, H., Nakajima, S. and Kobayashi, S. 1981. Tissue Antigens 18: 331-334.
306. Schauf, V., Ryan, S., Scollard, D., Jonasson, O., Brown, A., Nelson, K., Smith, T. and Vithayasai, V. 1985. Tissue Antigens 26: 243-247.
307. Van Eden, W., Mehra, N.K., Vaidya, M.C., D'Amaro, J., Schreuder, G.M.Th. and Van Rood, J.J. 1981. Tissue Antigens 18: 189-193.
308. De Vries, R.R.P., Mehra, N.K., Vaidya, M.C., Gupte, M.D., Meera Khan, P. and Van Rood, J.J. 1980. Tissue Antigens 16: 294-304.
309. Van Eden, W., De Vries, R.R.P., Mehra, N.K., Vaidya, M.C., D'Amaro, J. and Van Rood, J.J. 1980. J. Infect. Dis. 141: 693-701.
310. Xu, K., Fei, H., Su, B., Cao, J. et al. 1983. Chin. J. Dermatol. 16: 24-27.
311. Pollack, M.S., Ching, C., Pandey, J. and Reichert, E. 1985. Disease Markers 3: 119-129.
312. De Vries, R.R.P., Serjeantson, S.W. and Layrisse, Z. 1984. In: Histocompatibility Testing 1984. (Eds. Albert, E.D., Baur, M.P. and Mayr, W.R.) Springer Verlag, Heidelberg, pp. 362-367.

313. De Vries, R.R.P., Lai A Fat, R.F.M., Nijenhuis, L.E. and Van Rood, J.J. 1976. Lancet ii: 1328-1330.
314. Fine, P.E.M., Wolf, E., Pritchard, J., Watson, B., Bradley, D.J., Festeinstein, H. and Chacko, G.J.G. 1979. J. Infect. Dis. 140: 152-161.
315. Serjeantson, S.W. 1983. Immunol. Rev. 70: 24-47.
316. Van Eden, W., Gonzalez, N.M., De Vries, R.R.P., Convit, J. and Van Rood, J.J. 1985. J. Infect. Dis. 151: 9-14
317. Xu, K., De Vries, R.R.P., Fei, H., Van Leeuwen, A., Chen, R., and Ye, G. 1985. Int. J. Lepr. 53: 56-63.
318. Van Eden, W. and De Vries, R.R.P. 1984. Lepr. Rev. 55: 89-104.
319. Ottenhoff, T.H.M., Elferink, D.G., Hermans, J. and De Vries, R.R.P. 1985. Human Immunol. 13: 105-116.
320. Ottenhoff, T.H.M., Gonzalez, N.M., De Vries, R.R.P., Convit, J. and Van Rood, J.J. 1984. Tissue Antigens 24: 25-29.
321. Ottenhoff, T.H.M., Converse, P.J., Bjune, G. and De Vries, R.R.P. Submitted for publication.

CHAPTER 3

HLA CLASS-II-RESTRICTED *MYCOBACTERIUM LEPRAE*-REACTIVE T-CELL CLONES FROM LEPROSY PATIENTS ESTABLISHED WITH A MINIMAL REQUIREMENT FOR AUTOLOGOUS MONONUCLEAR CELLS*

Human helper T-cell clones (TLC) are exquisite tools for obtaining detailed information about which foreign antigenic epitopes and HLA class II restriction determinants are co-recognized by the T-cell receptor (reviewed in Ref. 15). Different techniques for generating TLC have been described, of which cloning under limiting dilution conditions has received most attention (15). For human antigen-specific helper TLC, the requirement for autologous or HLA class II identical antigen- presenting cells (APC) is well documented (see, for example, Refs 3, 4, 17 and 19).

One of the major obstacles in cloning T lymphocytes is the limited availability of autologous -or alternatively class II identical peripheral blood mononuclear cells (PBL)- especially from patients. These cells are continuously necessary for the restimulation of established TLC. A second problem is the generation of large numbers of cells from an individual TLC which would permit extensive functional and biochemical characterization. Recently, it has been shown that autologous Epstein- Barr-virus transformed B cells (EBV-BC) are capable of presenting foreign antigens such as tetanus toxoid and Mycobacterium leprae to T-cell lines and TLC (1, 5, 7, 13). The advantage of using EBV-BC as APC is that they provide a continuous and unlimited source of APC. Therefore we adapted and modified a recently described method (22) for the generation of TLC by using autologous EBV-BC as APC.

We have succeeded in generating TLC from three leprosy patients with a minimal requirement for autologous PBL. Our results demonstrate that these M. leprae-reactive TLC are HLA class II restricted and display strikingly different antigen recognition patterns: one TLC exclusively recognizes M. leprae and therefore may be M. leprae specific, two other TLC crossreact weakly with only one other mycobacterium, whereas a fourth TLC recognizes a determinant present on nearly all the mycobacteria tested.

* J.B.A.G. Haanen, T.H.M. Ottenhoff, A. Voordouw, B.G. Elferink, P.R. Klatser, H. Spits & R.R.P. de Vries. Scand. J. Immunol. v. 23: 101-108, 1986.

MATERIALS AND METHODS

Cells. PBL were isolated from heparinized venous blood by Ficoll- Isopaque density centrifugation (specific gravity, 1.077 g/ml, washed three times in Hanks' balanced salt solution (Gibco, Scotland, UK), and resuspended in Iscove's modified Dulbecco's medium (IMDM) (Gibco) supplemented with streptomycin (100 ug/ml), penicillin (100 U/ml) (both Flow Laboratories, Scotland, UK) and 10% pooled human AB serum (HS).

EBV-BC lines were generated from 5x106 autologous PBL as described previously (20).

The cells were frozen in 1 ml ampoules (Nunc, Roskilde, Denmark) containing 1-5x106 cells, 70% RPMI 1640 (Gibco), 20% screened pooled human AB plasma and 10% dimethylsulphoxide, and stored at -196°C.

Antigens. M. leprae antigens were kindly provided by Dr. M. Abe (National Institute of Leprosy Research, Tokyo, Japan) and the late Dr. C.C. Shepard (Centre for Infectious Diseases, Center for Disease Control, Atlanta, Ga, USA). Both preparations consisted of bacilli that were isolated from human lepromas according to Dharmendra's procedure (2) with slight modifications.

Sonicates of different mycobacteria including M. leprae purified from infected armadillo tissue were prepared by one of us (P.R.K.) as described in Ref. 10. Purified protein derivative (PPD) was obtained from the Staten Serum Institute (Copenhagen, Denmark).

Interleukin 2 (IL-2) containing supernatant. IL-2 containing supernatant (IL-2 sup) was kindly provided by Dr. L. Aarden (Central Laboratory of the Netherlands Red Cross Blood Transfusion Service, Amsterdam). The preparation is described in Ref. 14.

Antigen reactivation of PBL. PBL (5x106) of two tuberculoid (BC and R) and one borderline lepromatous leprosy patient (SC) were restimulated in vitro with M. leprae in IMDM supplement with 10% HS. The cultures were incubated for 5 days in 24-well tissue culture trays (Falcon 3047, Becton and Dickinson, Oxnard, Calif. USA) at 37°C in a fully humidified 5% CO2-air mixture.

Cloning of M. leprae-reactive T lymphoblasts (see Fig. 1). Enrichment of T-cell blasts was obtained either by Percoll (Pharmacia Fine Chemicals, Uppsala, Sweden) density centrifugation (12) or by continuing the cultures for another 3-10 days in the presence of 10% IL-2 sup (16). After the isolation of the blasts, a cell suspension was made containing 5 blasts/ml in a mixture consisting of (i) PBL from three or four random donors (106 cells/ml, 30 Gy irradiated), (ii) autologous EBV-BC (105 cells/ml, 50 Gy irradiated), and (iii) an optimal concentration of M. leprae antigen, all in IMDM supplemented with 10% HS. This suspension was plated in 96-well flat-bottom microtitre plates (Falcon 3072, Becton and Dickinson) (0.1 ml per well, i.e. 0.5 T lymphoblasts per well) and incubated as described above. The cultures were first screened for growth by light microscopy after 7-10 days. Growing cultures were transferred to 24-well tissue culture trays and restimulated with 1 ml per well of the cell-antigen mixture described above. Three to 4 days later, exogenous IL-2 sup (5%) was added. After an additional 4-7 days, the cultures were restimulated again until a minimum of 2x106 cells per culture was obtained.

The cells were frozen 3-8 days after the final restimulation. M. leprae-reactive TLC were further increased by restimulation as described above for 4 days, except that Leuko Agglutinine (Pharmacia Fine Chemicals, Sweden) was added to the cell antigen mixture (final concentration 1 ug/ml) in order to increase the yield of cells. This was followed by culturing for 3 days in the presence of IL-2 sup (5%).

Proliferation assays. 1x104 TLC (0.05 ml) and 5x104 irradiated (40 Gy) autologous or allogeneic PBL as AOC (0.05 ml) in IMDM with 10% HS were cultured with 0.1 ml of M. leprae antigen suspension in optimal concentration (4 ug/ml), or Dharmendra (Center for Disease Control), (1:120 dilution), in 96-well flat-bottom microtitre plates (Greiner, FRG). Phytohaemagglutinin (PHA) (Wellcome Diagnostics, Beckenham, Kent, UK: 4 ug/ml) and plain IMDM were used as control antigens. The cultures were set up in duplicate or triplicate and incubated as described above for 72 h. Eighteen hours before termination, 1.0 uCi of (3H) thymidine ((3H) TdR) (specific activity 6.7 Ci/mmol; Radiochemical Centre, Amersham, Bucks., UK)in 0.05 ml RPMI 1640 was added. The samples were harvested on glass-fibre filters using a semi-automatic sample harvester. (3H) TdR incorporation was assessed by counting in a liquid scintillation counter (Searle, Nuclear, Chicago, Ill., USA). All cells had been HLA typed as mentioned in Ref. 16.

Cell surface markers. Cell surface labelling was measured by a standard indirect immunofluorescence technique. The monoclonal antibodies used were OKT3 (Ortho Diagnostic Systems, Raritan, N.J., USA), RIV-6 (anti-T4, National Institute of Public Health, Bilthoven, The Netherlands) FK 18 (anti-T8, F. Koning, ref. 11). OK Ia1 (anti-Ia, Ortho), anti HLA-DR (Becton and Dickinson) and Leu 7 (Becton and Dickinson, recognizing a human natural killer cell-like determinant) all diluted from pure ascites. TLC were resuspended in PBS/1% BSA (106 cells/ml), divided into aliquots of 2.5x105 cells and labelled with 20 ul monoclonal antibody solution for 30 min at 0°C.

The cells were subsequently washed twice, incubated with goat anti-mouse immunoglobulin conjugated with fluorescein isothiocyanate (GAM/Ig/FITC) (Becton and Dickinson) for another 30 min at 0°C, and then rewashed.

GAM/Ig/FITC without monoclonal antibody was used as a control. Cells were analysed (104 per sample) in a fluorescence-activated cell sorter TM analyser (Becton and Dickinson).

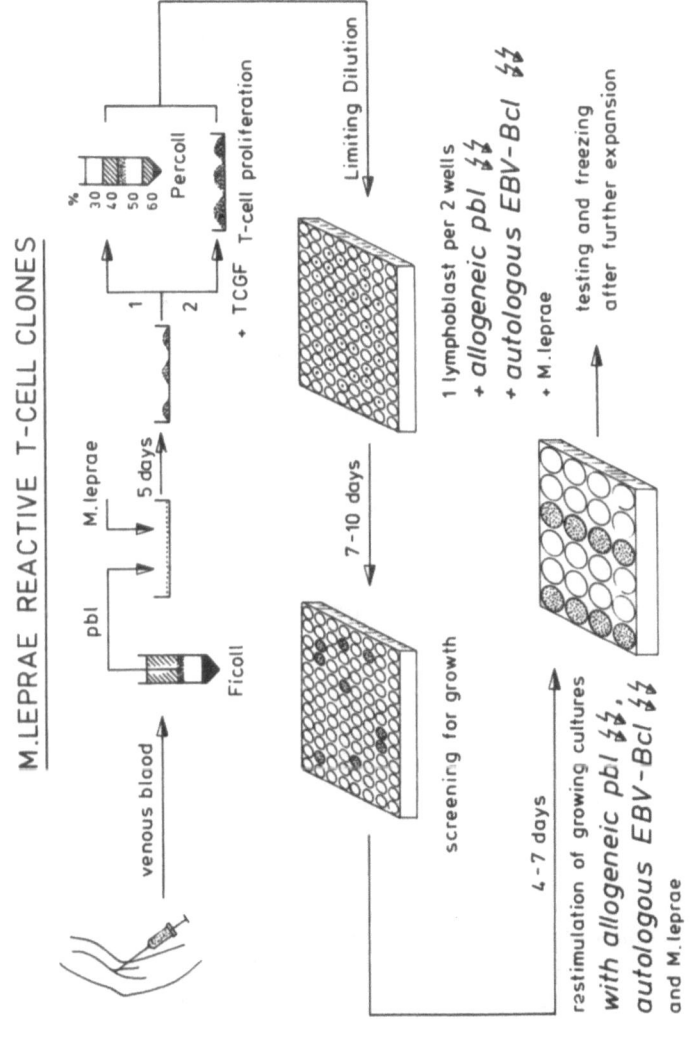

M.LEPRAE REACTIVE T-CELL CLONES

Fig. 1.

RESULTS

Cloning, long-term culture and enhancement of M. leprae responsiveness of TLC

During the first screening for growth by light microscopy adequate growth was observed in 60 cultures (28%) from patient BC, 49 (30%) from patient SC, and 56 (19%) from patient R. Upon further expansion only six (10%), three (6%), and zero (0%) clones respectively were lost. In the first screening for responsive TLC, in which M. leprae was presented by autologous APC, four TLC from patient BC, 13 TLC from patient SC and 34 TLC from patient R showed proliferative responses to M. leprae, ranging from 1200 to 32,000 cpm (data not shown). Most of these TLC could be restimulated and expanded several times as described above without losing their ability to proliferate towards M. leprae antigens presented by autologous or HLA class-II-compatible APC. So far we have expanded the majority of the TLC to actual numbers of more than 108 cells.

Interestingly, after further expansion of the four TLC of BC and the addition of exogenous IL-2 sup, a striking enhancement of M. leprae responsiveness was observed in comparison with the first M. leprae- directed proliferative responses (see Table I): proliferative responses showed a fivefold to twentyfold increase, whereas responses induced by PHA showed an increase of less than twofold. Consequently, we expanded and tested five other originally negative TLC from patient BC. Three of these five TLC then showed clear M. leprae reactivity, whereas the other two TLC remained non-responsive. A similar but less spectacular enhancement of M. leprae responsiveness was observed in some TLC from patients SC and R (data not shown).

Cell surface marker phenotypes of M. leprae-reactive TLC

The cell surface phenotypes of the tested responsive TLC were all T3, T4 OKIa1, HLA-DR positive and T8, Leu 7 negative.

HLA class II restriction of TLC responses towards M. leprae.

The HLA class II restriction of the TLC responses of patient BC towards M. leprae was investigated by presenting M. leprae via a selected panel of allogeneic irradiated APC, matched or mismatched with the class II antigens of BC as described in Ref. 16.

The class II phenotype of BC is DR3,4, DRw52,53, DQw3, DPw1,5. The results obtained with three TLC are shown in Table II. TLC VI 1E8 responds only to M. leprae in the presence of two out of nine DR4-positive APC, whereas TLC VI 5E7 responds in four out of eight DR4-positive APC, including the two recognized by VI 1E8.

TLC II 2F10 can only be activated by some but not all DR3-positive APC. The bulk T-cell line responds to M. leprae in the presence of all DR-shared APC except one DR-mismatched but DRw53- and DQw3-shared APC (data not shown). These results strongly suggest that these TLC co- recognize M. leprae only in association with HLA-DR-associated class II determinants.

Antigen specificity of four TLC from patient BC.

To determine the extent of specificity for M. leprae of four random TLC from patient BC, a panel of mycobacterial antigens was presented to these TLC. All four TLC react against three different M. leprae antigens, one of which is derived from human lepromas whereas the other two are different fractions from an ultrasonicate of armadillo-derived M. leprae bacilli (10). Therefore trivial explanations such as reactivity against human -or armadillo- tissue materials can be excluded. TLC VI 5E7 reacts with virtually all mycobacterial antigens and thus seems to recognize a common mycobacterial determinant. TLC VI 4F3 in contrast exclusively recognizes M. leprae antigens.

TLC II 2F10 reacts with M. leprae and weakly with M. tuberculosis, whereas TLC II 4A4 is activated strongly by M. leprae and weakly by M. kansasii.

DISCUSSION

In this report we describe M. leprae-reactive TLC (T3 + T4 + T8) from leprosy patients, generated by an effective method which minimizes the requirement for autologous PBL, i.e. 107 cells, which are present in approximately 10 ml of venous blood. TLC from one patient were characterized in more detail with respect to HLA class II restriction and M. lepraee specificity in their responses to M. leprae.

A major obstacle in the cloning of T lymphocytes from, in this case, leprosy patients is the limited availability of autologous mononuclear cells, which are needed for the continuous restimulation of these TLC (see, for example, Refs 3, 4, 17 and 19). Recently, however, several groups have shown that EBV-BC can present soluble antigens like tetanus toxoid to autologous TLC (1, 7, 13). Our group has demonstrated that EBV-BC are also capable of presenting M. leprae to M. leprae- reactive T-cell lines and TLC in an HLA-DR-restricted manner (5). The advantage of using EBV-BC as APC is (a) that they provide a continuous and unlimited source of autologous APC, and (b) that large numbers of antigen-reactive TLC cells can be obtained (108), thus allowing for extensive functional and biochemical studies. This may have important practical implications for studying among other things the HLA class II determinants and foreign antigenic epitopes recognized by T cells and their possible relation to disease.

We therefore modified and adapted a recently described method (22) for the cloning of T lymphocytes by using autologous EBV-BC as APC. Here we describe the method and show that M. leprae-reactive TLC can be generated and continuously restimulated with a minimal requirement for autologous PBL.

The enhancement in antigen responsiveness of several TLC during the extension of their culturing period is a remarkable finding, which has considerable implications for the screening of TLC for antigen responsiveness. This observation may reflect differences in the expression of the T-cell receptor (6), IL-2 receptors, or other functional determinants. Whatever its mechanism, it is important to note that an event dependent on cell cycle or differentiation stage may turn initially nonresponsive TLC into antigen-responsive TLC.

These M. leprae-reactive TLC are restricted by class II epitopes associated with but not identical to DR. These findings are in agreement with data from Qvigstad et al. (18), who have shown that DR4-associated restriction epitopes are associated with one of the five cellularly defined Dw subtypes within DR4 rather than with DR4 itself. Our results further show that two TLC apparently recognize two different types of DR4-associated restriction epitopes. Studies defining the fine specificity of the restriction epitopes used by these and several other TLC are in progress.

Finally, the four tested TLC from patient BC show a striking difference in the recognition of mycobacterial antigens. One TLC only recognizes M. leprae antigens and therefore may be M. leprae specific. So far, M. leprae-reactive TLC from immunized mice have displayed cross-reactivity against different mycobacteria (8, 9) like TLC VI 5E7 (Fig. 2).

Thus, T cells derived from leprosy patients may recognize antigenic determinants on M. leprae other than murine T cells. Since the DNA of M. leprae has now been cloned (21) it will soon become feasible to transcribe large quantities of M. leprae-specific proteins. These TLC will be important reagents in defining which M. leprae antigens are recognized by T cells and T-cell subsets, and will therefore be relevant for the development of a successful M. leprae vaccine (23).

ACKNOWLEDGEMENTS

The authors thank Dr. D.L. Leiker for his most helpful collaboration in obtaining blood from leprosy patients, Wim van Schooten for excellent technical assistance, Ruud Schuurman and Margriet Kraakman for establishing the autologous EBV-BC, and Joke Blom for assessing cell surface phenotypes; Annemarie Termijtelen for her critical and stimulating discussions, Joe D'Amaro for critically reading the manuscript and Ingrid Curiël for preparing this manuscript.

The investigations were supported (in part) by the Foundation for Medical Research FUNGO (Grant 13-83-01), the Immunology of Leprosy (IMMLEP)

59

component of the UNDP/World Bank/WHO Special Programme for Research and Training in Tropical diseases, and The Netherlands Leprosy Relief Association (NSL).

REFERENCES

1. Chu, E., Umetsu, D., Lareau, M., Scheeberger, E. & Geha, R.S. Analysis of antigen uptake and presentation by Epstein-Barr virus transformed lymphoblastoid B-cells. Eur. J. Immunol. 14, 291-298, 1984.
2. Dharmendra. Studies of the lepromin test. A bacillary antigen standardized by weight. Lepr. India 14, 122-129, 1942.
3. Eckels, D.D., Lake, P., Lamb, J.R., Johnsson, A.H., Shaw, S., Woody, J.N. & Hartzman, R.J. SB-restricted presentation of influenza and Herpes simplex virus antigens on human T lymphocyte clones. Nature 301, 716-718, 1983.
4. Eckels, D.D., Lamb, J.R., Lake P., Woody, J.N., Johnsson, A.H. & Hartzman, R.J. Antigen-specific human T lymphocyte clones. Genetic restriction of influenza virus-specific responses to HLA-D region genes. Human Immunol. 4, 313-324, 1982.
5. Elferink, B.G., Ottenhoff, T.H.M. & de Vries, R.R.P. Epstein-Barr virus-transformed B-cell lines present Mycobacterium leprae antigens to T cells. Scand. J. Immunol. 22, 585-590, 1985.
6. Haars, R., Rohowsky-Kochan, C., Reed, E., West King, D. & Suciu-Foca, N. Modulation of T-cell antigen receptor on lymphocyte membrane. Immunogenetics 20, 397-405, 1984.
7. Issekutz, T., Chu, E. & Geha, R.S. Antigen presentation by human B cells: T cell proliferation induced by Epstein-Barr virus B lymphoblastoid cells. J. Immunol. 129, 1446-1450, 1982.
8. Kaufmann, S.H.E. Biological activities of a murine T cell clone with reactivity to Mycobacterium leprae. Cell. Immunol. 83, 215-220, 1984.
9. Kingston, A.E. & Colston, M.J. Concentration-dependent effects of mycobacteria on the stimulation of murine T cell clones. Acta Leprologica 2, 369-377, 1984.
10. Klatser, P.R., van Rens, M.M. & Eggelte, T.A. Immunobiochemical characterization of Mycobacterium leprae antigens by the SDS-polyacrylamide gel electrophoresis immunoperoxidase technique (SGIP) using patient's sera. Clin. Exp. Immunol. 56, 537-544, 1984.
11. Koning, F., Kardol, M., van der Poel, J., Termijtelen, A., Goulmy, E., Ottenhoff, T., Blokland, E., Elferink, D., Pool, J., Naipal van den Berge, S. & Bruning, H. The influence of the workshop monoclonal antibodies on CML, AgTR, PLT, ADCC and NK-cell activity. In Reinherz, E.L. (ed.) Proc. 2nd Int. Workshop on Human Leucocyte Differentiation Antigens. Springer Verlag, Heidelberg (in press).
12. Kurnick, J.T., stberg, L., Stegagno, M., Kimura, A.K., in, A. & Sjöberg, O. A. rapid method for the separation of functional lymphoid cell populations of human and animal origin on PVP-silica (Percoll) density gradients. Scand. J. Immunol. 10, 563-573, 1979.
13. Lanzavecchia, A. Antigen specific interaction between T and B cells. Nature 314, 6011-6013, 1985.
14. Miedema, F., van Oostveen, J.W., Sauerwein, R.W., Terpstra, F.G., Aarden, L.A. & Melief, C.J.M. Induction of immunoglobulin synthesis by interleukin 2 is T4'/T8 cell dependent. A role for interleukin 2 in the pokeweed mitogen-driven system. Eur. J. Immunol. 15, 107-111, 1985.
15. Möller, G. T cell clones. Immun. Rev. 54, 1981.
16. Ottenhoff, T.H.M., Elferink, B.G., Hermans, J. & De Vries, R.R.P. HLA class II restriction repertoire of antigen specific T cells. I. The main restriction determinants for antigen presentation are associated with HLA-A/DR and not with DP and DQ. Human Immunol. 13, 105-116, 1985.
17. Qvigstad, E., Moen, T. & Thorsby, E. T cell clones with similar antigen specificity may be restricted by DR, MT (DC), or SB class II HLA molecules. Immunogenetics 19, 455-460, 1984.
18. Qvigstad, E., Scott, H. & Thorsby, E. HLA class-II restriction of antigen specific T cell

activation. Prog. Allergy 36, 73-94, 1985.

19. Sredni, B., Volkmann, D., Schwartz, R. & Fauci, A.S. Antigen specific human T cell clones: development of clones requiring HLA-DR compatible presenting cells for stimulation in presence of antigen. Proc. Nat. Acad. Sci. USA 78, 1858-1862, 1981.

20. Steinitz, M., Koshimies, S., Klein, G. & Mäkelä, O. Establishment of specific antibody producing human lines by antigen preselection and EBV transformation. Curr. Top. Microbiol. Immun. 81, 156, 1978.

21. Young, R.A., Mehra, V., Sweetser, D., Buchanan, T.M., Clark-Curtiss, J., Davis, R.W. & Bloom, B.R. Genes for the major protein antigens of the leprosy parasite Mycobacyterium leprae. Nature, Lond. 316, 450-452, 1985.

22. Yssel, H., de Vries, J.E., Koken, M., van Blitterswijk, W. & Spits, H. Serum-free medium for generation and propagation of functional human cytotoxic and helper T cell clones. J. Immun. Methods 72, 219-227, 1984.

23. Ottenhoff, T.H.M., Klatser, P.R., Ivanyi, J., Elferink, B.G., de Wit, M.Y.L. & de Vries, R.R.P. Mycobacterium leprae specific protein antigens defined by cloned human helper T cells. Nature (in press).

CHAPTER 4

MYCOBACTERIUM LEPRAE SPECIFIC PROTEIN ANTIGENS DEFINED BY CLONED HUMAN HELPER T CELLS *

Leprosy displays a remarkable spectrum of symptoms correlating with the T cell mediated immune reactivity of the host against the causative organism, *Mycobacterium leprae* (1). At one pole of this spectrum are lepromatous leprosy patients showing a *M. leprae* specific T cell unresponsiveness (2); at the other pole are tuberculoid leprosy patients displaying both acquired immunity and delayed type hypersensitivity against *M. leprae* which are thought to be conferred by helper T (Th) cells (1,3–5). Because well defined *M. leprae* antigens are crucial for the prevention and the control of leprosy (1,6,7), we have cloned *M. leprae* reactive T cells (TLC) of the helper phenotype from a tuberculoid leprosy patient. As reported here, these TLC show an unexpected diversity in the recognition of *M. leprae* and related mycobacteria, which is different from that exhibited by monoclonal antibodies (8,9). Half of these TLC are completely or almost *M. leprae* specific, whereas the other half is crossreactive with most or all other mycobacteria. A *M. leprae* protein of relative molecular mass (M_r) 36,000 (36K) defined by a *M. leprae* specific monoclonal antibody (7,8,10) stimulates 4 out of 6 TLC tested. Each of these TLC recognizes a different antigenic determinant, one of which is *M. leprae* specific.

Whereas the *M. leprae* specific unresponsiveness in lepromatous leprosy patients may be triggered by specific immunosuppression inducing determinants on the bacillus (11), virtually nothing is known about the antigens recognized by Th cells responsible for the cell-mediated immune reactivity against *M. leprae* in tuberculoid leprosy patients. To study the antigenic determinants involved in activating these T cells in more detail, we have cloned *M. leprae* reactive T cells of a tuberculoid leprosy patient.

Peripheral blood mononuclear cells of a tuberculoid leprosy patient were restimulated *in vitro* with *M. leprae* antigen, cloned and propagated as described elsewhere (12). Autologous Epstein–Barr virus transformed B cells (EBV-BC) were used as antigen presenting cells (APC) as evidence suggests that these cells can effectively present *M. leprae* antigens to primed T cells (for review see ref. 13). One advantage of using EBV-BC as APC is that such cells provide a continuous

*Tom H.M. Ottenhoff, Paul R. Klatser, Juraj Ivanyi, Diënne G. Elferink, Madeleine Y.L. de Wit and René R.P. de Vries, 1986. Nature 319: 66–68.

and unlimited source of APC, which drastically reduces the number of autologous peripheral blood mononuclear cells needed for the cloning and propagation of antigen specific T cells.

Twenty-three *M. leprae* reactive proliferative TLC were selected at random and studied in more detail with regard to their antigen specificity. All 23 TLC were of the $CD3^+CD4^+CD8^-$ phenotype, and were strongly positive for HLA-DR. Twenty-two TLC were restricted in their response by HLA-DR determinants and one by an hitherto unknown polymorphic HLA-DQ determinant, as assessed by panel and inhibition studies (see chapter 5).

Two *M. leprae* preparations of different origin, ultrasonicates from 19 other mycobacteria, and the purified protein derivative (PPD) of *M. tuberculosis* were presented to these TLC via autologous or HLA class II compatible APC. The results shown in figure 1 reveal four patterns of antigen reactivity :a) TLC recognizing determinants exclusively expressed by *M. leprae* (n = 6), b) TLC activated by determinants present on *M. leprae* and crossreactive with one or two other mycobacterial strains, mainly *M. vaccae* and *M. lepraemurium* (n = 5), c) TLC reactive with several but not all mycobacteria (n = 2) and d) TLC triggered by crossreactive determinants present on all mycobacteria, sometimes with the exception of *M. nonchromogenicum* (n = 10). None of the TLC showed proliferative responses in the presence of APC and either tetanus toxoid or *Candida albicans*, which represented non-mycobacterial control antigens. Similar data were obtained with TLC from another tuberculoid patient (data not shown).

Recently, five *M. leprae* proteins have been described that contain *M. leprae* specific antigens recognized by murine monoclonal antibodies (7–9,14). The M_r's of these proteins are 12K, 18K, 28K, 36K and (55-) 65K. To investigate whether these antibody defined *M. leprae* proteins are also recognized by human T cells, we tested the 12K and 36K *M. leprae* proteins which had been purified by using respectively the *M. leprae* specific monoclonal antibodies ML06A1 (refs. 8,9) and F47-9-1 (refs. 8,10). Six different *M. leprae* reactive TLC, and a *M. leprae*-generated polyclonal T lymphoblast culture (T-LB) (15) from the same patient (T-LB1) and from a second tuberculoid leprosy patient (T-LB2) were tested.

The data presented in Table 1 show that the *M. leprae* specific 36K protein is recognized by four out of the six TLC tested and both T-LB, whereas the *M. leprae* specific 12K purified protein is recognized only by one TLC and (weakly) by one T-LB, each of which is also reactive with the 36K protein. As all four TLC reacting with the 36K protein display different antigen-specificity patterns (figure 1), they must recognize four different antigenic determinants on the 36K protein, only one of which is clearly *M. leprae* specific. The finding that only one of the two *M. leprae* specific TLC (1E4) recognized the 36K protein suggests that the other *M. leprae* specific TLC tested (1G5) reacts with another *M. leprae* specific determinant not expressed on the 36K protein. In addition, as only one of the two completely crossreactive TLC (3E8) tested reacts with the 36K protein, at least two common mycobacterial determinants are defined by these TLC, one of which resides on the 36K protein.

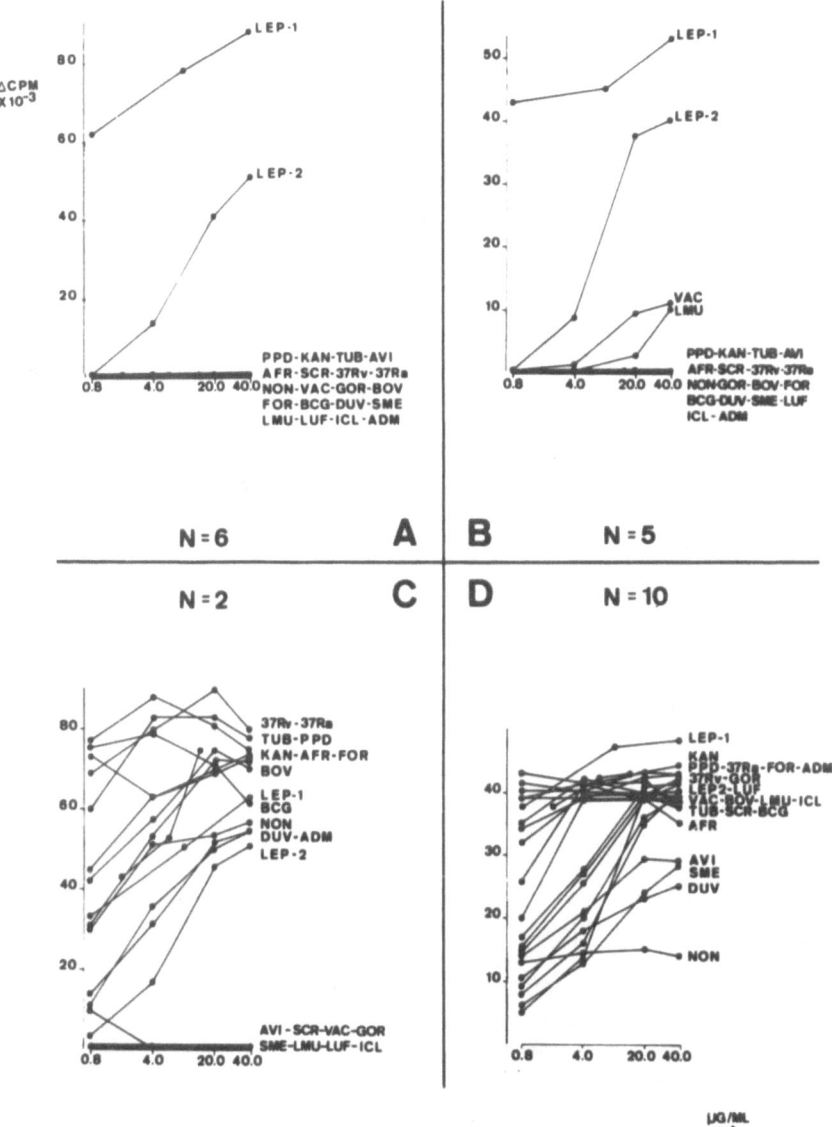

Fig. 1

Antigen specificity of *Mycobacterium leprae* reactive cloned T cells.

Mycobacterial antigens were presented via autologous or HLA class II compatible APC to 23 different *M. leprae* reactive TLC from a tuberculoid leprosy patient. The antigens tested were: LEP-1: Dharmendra lepromin, consisting of bacilli isolated from human lepromas; LEP-2: armadillo derived *M. leprae*; PPD: purified protein derivative of *M. tuberculosis* (obtained from Statens Serum

Institute, Copenhagen); KAN: *M. kansasii*; TUB: *M. tuberculosis*; AVI: *M. avium*; AFR: *M. africanum*; SCR: *M. scrofulaceum*; 37Rv: *M. tuberculosis H37Rv*; 37Ra: *M. tuberculosis H37Ra*; NON: *M. nonchromogenicum*; VAC: *M. vaccae*; GOR: *M. gordonae*; BOV: *M. bovis*; FOR: *M. fortuitum*; BCG: *M. bovis BCG*; DUV: *M. duvalii*; SME: *M. smegmatis*; LMU: *M. lepraemurium*; LUF: *M. lufu*; ICL: *M. avium intracellulare*; ADM: armadillo derived aspecific mycobacteria. Dharmendra lepromin was tested in dilutions of 1:240, 1:120 and 1:60; PPD was tested in concentrations of 1.7, 5.0 and 16.7 μg/ml. All other mycobacteria had been ultrasonicated as described in ref. 21, and were tested at 0.8, 4.0, 20.0 and 40.0 μg/ml. Four different reactivity patterns were observed (A-D), and a representative example of each pattern is shown. Results are expressed as mean Δ counts per minute x 10^{-3} (^{3}H-thymidine incorporation) of duplicate cultures (standard deviations in most cases were less than 10%) as assessed by substracting background proliferation in the absence of antigen from responses in the presence of antigen.

Methods

Antigen reactivation, cloning, expansion and proliferative assays were performed as described elsewhere (12). Briefly, peripheral blood mononuclear cells were isolated by Ficoll-Isopaque density centrifugation and restimulated *in vitro* with an optimal concentration of Dharmendra lepromin (1:120 - 1:60) in 24 well tissue culture trays. T cell blasts, enriched for by Percoll density centrifugation, were then cloned by limiting dilution in a feeder cell mixture consisting of irradiated autologous EBV-BC (10^5 cells ml^{-1}), peripheral blood mononuclear cells of 3–4 random donors (10^6 cells ml^{-1}), and Dharmendra lepromin (1:120 - 1:60). Of the originally 295 microwells seeded, 56 contained growing cultures and 34 of these showed proliferative responses. Growing cultures were restimulated once a week with the feeder mixture, supplemented with Leuko Agglutinin A(1 μg ml^{-1}) (Pharmacia, Sweden) and expanded in the presence of interleukin-2 containing supernatants. In proliferative assays, 10^4 TLC and $5x10^4$ irradiated autologous or HLA class II compatible peripheral blood mononuclear cells as APC and antigen were co-cultured in flat-bottomed 96-well microtitre plates (Greiner, FRG). After 72 hours, 1.0 μCi ^{3}H-thymidine was added to each well. Cultures were harvested 16 hours later on glass-fibre filters using a semi automatic sample harvester. ^{3}H-thymidine incorporation was assessed by liquid scintillation counting.

The six TLC an the two T-LB have so far failed to respond to 3,6-di-0-methylglucose-$(CH_2)_8$-bovine serum albumin, when tested at a wide range of concentrations (5.10^{-3}–2.10^3 μgml^{-1}). This synthetic antigen contains a *M. leprae* specific monosaccharide component which forms the terminal part of the trisaccharide complex on *M. leprae* phenolic glycolipid. This gyclolipid has been shown to trigger *M. leprae* specific suppressor T cells in lepromatous but not in tuberculoid patients, as measured by inhibition of concanavalin-A stimulated peripheral blood mononuclear cell cultures (13).

Thus, 6 out of 23 human helper TLC recognized at least two separate determinants that are uniquely expressed by *M. leprae*, but which are distinct from those defined by murine monoclonal antibodies, only a few of which have been found to recognize *M. leprae* specific protein antigens (7–10,14). So far, all murine *M. leprae* reactive TLC crossreact with other mycobacteria (16,17). The finding that 3 out of 5 nearly *M. leprae* specific human TLC also react with *M. vaccae* is in accord with the results of *in vivo* skin tests which revealed a selective crossreactivity between *M. leprae* and *M. vaccae* (18).

Table 1
M. leprae-specific and crossreactive TLC recognize different determinants on a M. leprae-specific monoclonal antibody

Antigen	T cell: Antigen specificity:	IG5 LEP (a)*	1E4 LEP (a)	2F9 LEP- VAC- LMU (b)	3B4 Partly cross- reactive (c)	1F9 Completely cross- reactive (d)	3E8 Completely cross- reactive (d)	TLB1	TLB2
M. leprae		14.2 ± 4.3	57.9 ± 0.1	88.4 ± 6.2	42.2 ± 2.1	10.0 ± 2.0	70.5 ± 3.5	53.7 ± 5.0	46.7 ± 0.9
36K M. leprae protein		0.1 ± 0.0	24.0 ± 5.5	26.8 ± 0.5	21.4 ± 0.6	0.2 ± 0.0	20.0 ± 0.2	18.2 ± 4.9	17.2 ± 3.4
12K M. leprae protein		0.1 ± 0.1	0.1 ± 0.0	48.8 ± 5.4	0.2 ± 0.1	0.1 ± 0.0	5.9 ± 1.4	0.2 ± 0.0	3.9 ± 0.9
Medium		0.0 ± 0.0	0.1 ± 0.1	0.1 ± 0.1	0.2 ± 0.1	0.1 ± 0.0	2.3 ± 1.8	0.1 ± 0.1	0.3 ± 0.0

The results are expressed as the mean $cpm \times 10^{-3} \pm$ S.D. of duplicate cultures. Positive cultures are boxed and are defined as exceeding the mean background proliferation with at least 3 S.D. and in addition given $> 10^3$ cpm. Proliferation assays were carried out as described in the legend of Fig. 1. M. leprae antigen is Dharmendra lepromin. The 36K protien was purified by the fast protein liquid chromatography system (FPLC; Pharmacia, Sweden). Briefly, M. leprae sonicate was applied on an anion-exchange column (Mono Q, HR5/5, Pharmacia, Sweden) and eluted with a linear salt gradient. Further purification was carried out on a gel permeation column (TSK G3000SW, LKB, Sweden). The purity of the antigen was analysed by SDS-polyacrylamide gel electrophoresis and SDS-polyacrylamide gel electrophoresis immunoperioxidase assay (21). The 12K protein was purified by affinity chromatography using monoclonal antibody ML06A1 coupled to cyanogen bromide-activated Sepharose 4B, followed by elution with 3M NaSCN (9). The optimal stimulatory concentration for the 36K protein was $16 \mu g$ ml^{-1}, and for the 12K protein $0,4 \mu g$ ml^{-1}. T.LB1 are polyclonal T lymphoblasts from the same patient, T-LB2 from a second tuberculoid leprosy patient, generated as described in ref 15.

* for abbreviations see legend figure 1.

The TLC described in this paper define antigenic determinants on purified *M. leprae* proteins capable of triggering T cells. It remains to be elucidated which *M. leprae* antigenic determinants recognized by these helper TLC are involved in protective immunity as opposed to immunopathology. A comparison of the antigenic determinants defined by TLC from healthy contacts with those defined by TLC from tuberculoid leprosy patients may be helpful in distinguishing between the two groups of *M. leprae* antigens. In addition to these two groups, a third group of antigens may be involved in the induction of *M. leprae* specific suppression (6,11). Recently, we have cloned *M. leprae* reactive suppressor T cells. Thus, we will be able to study whether different antigenic determinants are recognized by cloned helper and suppressor T cells.

Thus the use of TLC and purified *M. leprae* proteins will enable us to define the *M. leprae* antigens involved in T cell mediated protective immunity, immunopathology and possibly suppression; these, therefore, are exquisite tools for the rational design of a *M. leprae* vaccine and skin test reagents (1,6).

The T cell responses against these proteins cannot be inhibited by the relevant monoclonal antibodies (data not shown); this was not unexpected because, as a rule, antibodies and T cells react with different epitopes of the same antigen (see, for example, ref. 19). It is interesting that four out of the six TLC and both T-LB react with the 36K protein whereas only one of these TLC and one T-LB respond to one of the four other *M. leprae* proteins known – that is, the 12K protein. This result suggests that Th cells preferentially recognize immunodominant antigenic determinants (20) expressed on the 36K protein. Recently, the genes for the major proteins of *M. leprae* have been cloned and expressed (7) and indeed the five above mentioned *M. leprae* specific proteins have been found. Therefore, it should now be possible to determine whether one or more of the antigenic determinants on the 36K protein are formed – in part– by lipid or carbohydrate components.

We thank Dr. R.J.W. Rees and the late Dr. C.C. Shepard for providing us with *M. leprae* antigens; Dr. D.L. Leiker for his help in obtaining blood samples from leprosy patients; Arend Kolk and Frits Koning for monoclonal antibodies; Teunis Eggelte for synthetic saccharide antigens; John Haanen and Earl Johanns for technical assistance and Tiny van Westerop for drawing part of the figure and preparing the manuscript. This study was supported in part by the Foundation for Medical Research FUNGO (grant nr. 13-83-01), the Immunology of Leprosy (IMMLEP) component of the UNDP/WORLD Bank/WHO Special Programme for Research and Training in Tropical Diseases, and "the Netherlands Leprosy Relief Association (NSL)".

Note added in proof: Recent experiments show that also on the recombinant 36K *M. leprae* specific protein, expressed in *Escherichia coli*, different *M. leprae* specific protein determinants are detected by these *M. leprae* specific TLC.

References

1. Bloom, B.R. & Godal, T. Rev. Infect. Dis. 5, 765–780 (1983).
2. Bloom, B.R. & Mehra, V. Immunol. Rev. 80, 5–28 (1984).
3. Rees, R.J.W. Nature 211, 576 (1966).
4. Patel, P.J. & Lefford, M.J. Infect. Immun. 19, 87–93 (1978).
5. Lowe, C., Brett, S.J. & Rees, R.J.W. Clin. exp. Immunol. 61, 336–342 (1985).
6. Mitchison, N.A. Nature 308, 112–113 (1984).
7. Young, R.A., Mehra, V., Sweetser, D., Buchanan, T.M., Clark-Curtiss, J., Davis, R.W. & Bloom, B.R. Nature 316, 450–452 (1985).
8. Engers, H.D., Abe, M., Bloom, B.R., Mehra, V., Britton, W., Buchanan, T.M., Khanolkar, S.K., Young, D.B., Closs, O., Gillis, T., Harboe, M., Ivanyi, J., Kolk, A.H.J. & Shepard, C.C. Infect. Immunity 48, 603–605 (1985).
9. Ivanyi, J., Morris, J.A. & Keen, M. in: *Monoclonal antibodies Against Bacteria* (eds. Macario, A.J.L. & Macario, E.C.) (Academic Press, New York) (in press).
10. Klatser, P.R., de Wit, M.Y.L. & Kolk, A.H.J. Clin. exp. Immunol. 62, 468–473 (1985).
11. Mehra, V., Brennan, P.J., Rada, E., Convit,, J. & Bloom, B.R. Nature 308, 194–196 (1984).
12. Haanen, J.B.A.G., Ottenhoff, T.H.M., Voordouw, A., Elferink, D.G., Klatser, P.R., Spits, H. & de Vries, R.R.P. Scand. J. Immunol. 23, 101–108 (1986).
13. Elferink, B.G., Ottenhoff, T.H.M. & de Vries, R.R.P. Scand. J. Immunol. 22, 585–589 (1985).
14. Young, D.B., Fohn, M.J., Khanolkar, S.R. & Buchanan, T.M. Clin. exp. Immunol. 60, 546–552 (1985).
15. Ottenhoff, T.H.M., Elferink, B.G., Hermans, J. & de Vries, R.R.P. Human Immunol. 13, 105–116 (1985).
16. Kaufmann, S.H.E. Cell. Immunol. 83, 215–220 (1984).
17. Kingston, A.E. & Colston, M.J. Acta Leprologica 2, 369–377 (1984).
18. Stanford, J.L. in: *The Biology of the Mycobacteria* (eds. Ratledge, C. & Stanford, J.L.) Vol. 2, 85–127 (Academic Press, London) (1983).
19. Lamb, J.R., Eckels, D.D., Lake, P., Woody, J.N. & Green, N. Nature 300, 66–69 (1982).
20. Manca, F., Clarke, J.A., Miller, A., Sercarz, E.E. & Shastri, N.J. Immunol. 133, 2075–2078 (1984).
21. Klatser, P.R., van Rens, M.M. & Eggelte, T.A. Clin. exp. Immunol 56, 537–544 (1984).

CHAPTER 5

CLONED SUPPRESSOR T CELLS FROM A LEPROMATOUS LEPROSY PATIENT SUPPRESS *MYCOBACTERIUM LEPRAE* REACTIVE HELPER T CELLS*

Leprosy is a chronic infectious disease caused by *Mycobacterium leprae*. A characteristic feature of the disease is its remarkable spectrum of clinical symptoms correlating with the cellular immune responsiveness of the patient (1): at one pole of this spectrum are tuberculoid patients displaying both acquired cell-mediated immunity and delayed type hypersensitivity against the bacillus (2–4). At the other pole are lepromatous patients which show a specific T cell unresponsiveness against *M. leprae* (5). In between those two poles variable degrees of tuberculoid and lepromatous features may be seen in borderline leprosy patients. Thus far, studies on the mechanism of the antigen specific unresponsiveness in lepromatous leprosy have been contradictory and difficult to interpret, probably because of the use of heterogeneous cell populations in those experiments (6–10). We have now succeeded in cloning *M. leprae* stimulated T helper as well as T suppressor cells from a borderline lepromatous patient. The Ts clones of this patient specifically suppress responses of peripheral T cells as well as Th clones induced by both *M. leprae* and other mycobacteria, but not unrelated antigen or mitogen. These Ts cells also completely suppress Th cell responses against a *M. leprae* specific protein with a relative molecular mass of 36,000 (36K), suggesting the presence of a suppression inducing determinant on this 36K *M. leprae* protein.

In contrast to *M. leprae* activated and by interleukin-2 (IL–2) propagated T cell lines and clones derived from tuberculoid leprosy patients, similar T cell lines of (borderline) lepromatous leprosy patients consistently failed to show a proliferative response against *M. leprae* antigens presented by autologous or allogeneic HLA class II matched antigen presenting cells (APC) (data not shown). This lack of proliferation by cultured T cells to *M. leprae* was also observed when the peripheral blood mononuclear cells (PBMNC) of such (borderline) lepromatous patients did proliferate to *M. leprae*. We selected one such a borderline lepromatous patient whose peripheral T cells did proliferate against *M. leprae* as well as to unrelated antigens like herpes simplex virus (HSV) and mitogen (phytohaemagglutinin; PHA) because this might enable us to study both helper

*Tom H.M. Ottenhoff, Diënne G. Elferink, Paul R. Klatser and René R.P. de Vries. 1986. Nature 322: 462–464.

and possibly suppressor T cell responses against *M. leprae*. We then tested the *M. leprae* non responsive T cell line on autologous antigen activated peripheral T cells, thereby circumventing allogeneic effects. As shown in figure 1, the *M.*

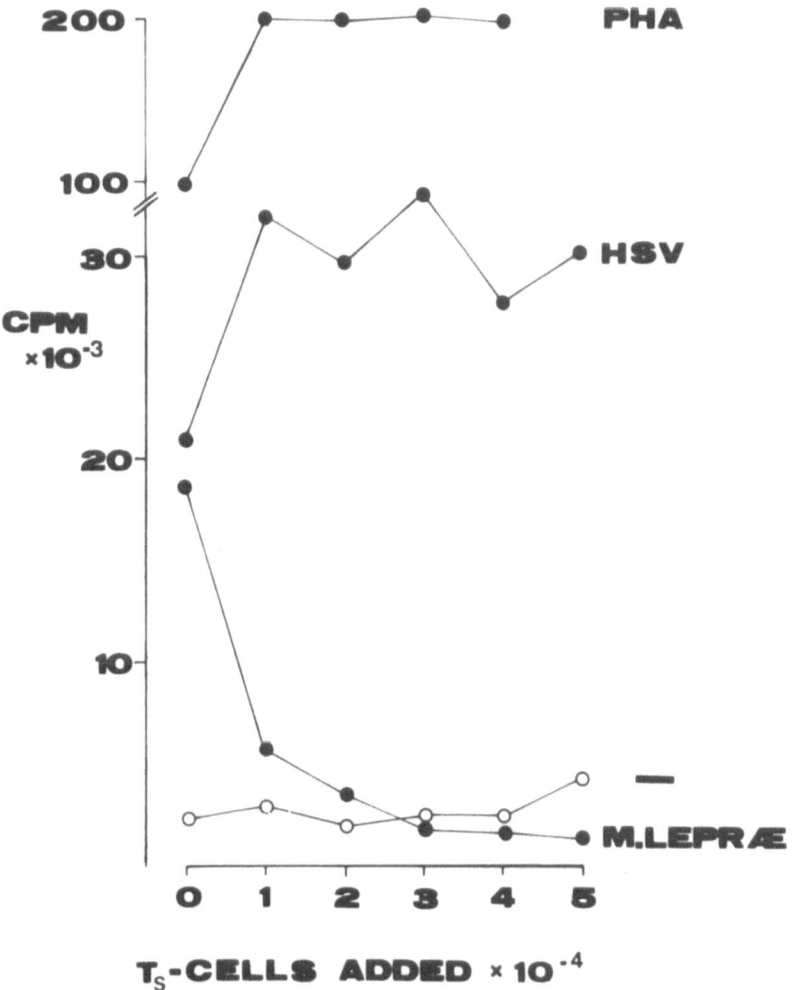

Fig. 1
Antigen specific suppression of *M. leprae* but not herpes simplex virus (HSV) or PHA induced proliferative peripheral T cell responses by a *M. leprae* induced and in IL-2 grown suppressor T cell line. The latter was added to 10^5 PBMNC in concentrations of 0, 1, 2, 3, 4 or 5 x 10^4 cells per culture. The results are expressed as the mean cpm of duplicate cultures (^{3}H-thymidine incorporation). Standard deviations mostly did not exceed 20%.
M. leprae antigens isolated from human lepromas and from armadillo infected tissue induced similar suppression.

Methods

PBMNC of a borderline lepromatous leprosy patient were isolated from heparinized venous blood by Ficoll-Isopaque density centrifugation (Pharmacy, University Hospital Leiden), washed three times in Hanks' balanced salt solution (Gibco, Scotland) and resuspended in Iscove's modified Dulbecco's medium (IMDM; Gibco) supplemented with 100 μg ml^{-1} streptomycin, 100 U ml^{-1} penicillin (both Flow Laboratories, Scotland) and 10% heat inactivated human AB serum. The diagnosis of this and other patients used for this study was based on regular clinical examination, lepromin skin test and skin biopsy histology by Dr. D.L. Leiker, Department of Dermatology, University Hospital of Amsterdam, the Netherlands. A standard lymphocyte transformation test was set up with 10^5 PBMNC per culture, to which antigen was added. The antigens tested were Dharmendra lepromin, consisting of bacilli isolated from human lepromas (obtained from the Centre for Infectious Diseases, Centres for Disease Control, Atlanta, U.S.A.; 1:80 dilution) and herpes simplex virus (obtained from the National Institute of Public Health, Bilthoven, The Netherlands; 1:64 dilution). From the start of the culture, either no or 1, 2, 3, 4 or 5 x 10^4 T cells of the nonresponsive T cell line (vide infra) were added to the culture. The cultures were set up in flat-bottomed 96-well microtitre plates (Greiner, FRG), incubated at 37 °C in a fully humidified 5% CO_2-air mixture for 5 days after which 1.0 μCi ^{3}H-thymidine was added to each well; the cultures were collected 16 hours later on glass-fibre filters using a semi-automatic sample harvester. ^{3}H-TdR incorporation was assessed by liquid scintillation counting.

The T cell line was generated as described previously (16,30). In brief, PBMNC were restimulated in vitro with an optimal concentration of Dharmendra lepromin (1:80) in 24-well tissue culture plates. T-cell blasts were then cultured for 10 days in the presence of 20% IL-2 containing medium (Lymfocult-T, Biotest, FRG). The cells were tested then for antigen induced proliferation in the presence of autologous APC and antigen but failed to show a response. The cells were then restimulated with a feeder mixture consisting of irradiated autologous EBV-BC as autologous APC (31) (10^5 cells ml^{-1}), PBMNC from 3-4 random donors (10^6 cells ml^{-1}) and Dharmendra lepromin (1:80). The cultures were further expanded in the presence of IL-2. The cells were then collected, tested again for non responsiveness against antigen and used for experiments. All cells were cultured in IMDM supplemented with 10% human AB serum.

leprae non responsive T cell line suppressed specifically and strongly M. leprae but not HSV or PHA responses. Peripheral responding T cells were mainly CD4 positive. The same result was obtained with 5 other M. leprae induced T cell lines of the same patient, all of which were antigen non responsive but IL-2 responsive.

Cloned T cells were derived from one such a line. None of these clones proliferated to M. leprae in the presence of APC, similar to the parental T cell line (data not shown). All these clones suppressed M. leprae but not HSV specific responses of peripheral T cells (table 1). Peripheral T cell responses against M. tuberculosis, M. fortuitum or PPD (purified protein derivative of M. tuberculosis) were also suppressed in variable degrees by these Ts clones. The cell surface marker phenotypes of the Ts cell line and Ts clones are also shown in table 1. All Ts clones were CD3 positive, confirming the T cell lineage nature of these cells. All Ts clones were also CD8 positive, whereas some showed a weak (1D8,1D11) or clear (1E9) double staining for CD4. The simultaneous expression of CD4 and CD8 by peripheral T cells and T cell clones has been reported

Table 1

Ts clones and line suppress the response of PBMNC to *M. Leprae* and other mycobacteria but not unrelated antigen.

Ts clone :	1D8	1D11	1E9	1D10	3D2	1G2	Ts line
CD phenotype:	4,8	4,8	4(8)	8	8	8	4,8
% suppression of response of PBMNC to:							
M. leprae	70	95	73	53	54	53	88
M. tuberculosis	24	55	70	44	39	n.t.	80
M. fortuitum	20	48	72	34	40	n.t.	91
PPD	2	44	56	50	50	n.t.	76
HSV	-250	12	-8	-231	-56	5	-59

The results are expressed as the percentage suppression of peripheral T cell responses against the respective antigens after the addition of 3×10^4 T suppressor cells, as calculated with the formula (1-cpm of peripheral T cells cultured in the presence of suppressor T cells/cpm of peripheral T cells in the absence of suppressor T cells) x 100%. Peripheral T cell responses in the absence of suppressor cells against *M. leprae* were: 21,920 cpm, against *M. tuberculosis*: 26,570, against *M. fortuitum*: 15,605, against PPD: 6,060 and against HSV: 29,300. Responses in the absence of antigen were 970 cpm. All results are given as the mean cpm of duplicate cultures. Standard deviations did not exceed 20%. The CD4,8 phenotypes of the T cell line and clones are shown. n.t. = not tested.

Methods

The cultures were set up as described in the legend of fig. 1. The antigens tested in addition were ultrasonicates of whole mycobacteria (20 μg ml^{-1}) and PPD (5.0 μg ml^{-1}). From the suppressor T cell line, clones were prepared by cloning the cells (1D8, 1D10, 1D11: 10 cells per well; 1E9, 3D2, 1G2; 0.5 cell per well) on the feeder cell mixture described in the legend of fig. 1, supplemented with Leuko Agglutinin A (1 μg ml^{-1}) (Pharmacia, Sweden) and expanding the cultures in the presence of exogenous IL-2. This cycle was repeated several times (see ref. 32). The cell surface marker phenotypes of the different T cells were determined by a standard indirect immunofluorescence technique as described in ref. 32. The monoclonal antibodies used were OKT3 (Ortho) for the CD3 marker, RIV-6 (anti-T4/leu 3; Nat. Inst. Public Health, Bilthoven, the Netherlands) for the CD4 marker, FK18 (anti-T8/leu2; gift of F. Koning) for the CD8 marker, B8.11.2 (anti HLA-DR; gift of B. Malissen), SPV-L3 (anti HLA-DQ; gift of H. Spits) and B7/21 (anti HLA-DP; gift of F. Bach) for respectively HLA-DR, DQ and DP antigens.

recently (11,12). The clones strongly expressed HLA-DR antigens whereas the expression of DQ and DP varied.

Recently the genes for the five major proteins of *M. leprae* have been cloned and expressed in *Escherichia coli* (13). One of these five proteins is a *M. leprae* specific 36K protein (13-15). This protein was recently shown to contain several different antigenic determinants capable of stimulating Th cells. These determinants include both *M. leprae* specific and crossreactive ones as defined by *M. leprae* specific and crossreactive Th clones from tuberculoid patients (16). Peripheral T cells of the suppressor cell donor reacted with this 36K protein. This offered us the possibility to ask the question whether these 36K reactive Th cells could be suppressed by the autologous Ts cells. A negative result would indicate that the epitope(s) recognized by Ts cells resides neither on the 36K protein nor on the 36K reactive Th cells, thus enabling us to dissociate easily the induction of *M. leprae* reactive Th and Ts. This is of course not only important for experimental purposes, but also for the prevention (vaccine) and maybe even therapy of leprosy. However, as shown in figure 2, the 36K response could be inhibited completely by the Ts cells. This result may indicate that the 36K protein in addition to helper epitopes also contains at least one suppressor epitope. This 36K epitope then would be the first *M. leprae* suppressor epitope on a *M. leprae* protein, because we consider it unlikely that the 36K protein would contain the *M. leprae* specific phenolic glycolipid, which has been reported to induce suppression of concanavalin-A stimulated PBMNC of lepromatous patients (5,7). The co-existence of both helper and suppressor epitopes on the 36K protein would closely resemble the situation for other immunogenic proteins like hen egg white lysozyme (17), β-galactosidase (18) and a 185K streptococcal protein (19). For the first two protein antigens it has been shown that the putative suppressor epitope has to be situated on the same molecule or fragment as the helper epitope in order to induce suppression of the immune response (20,21).

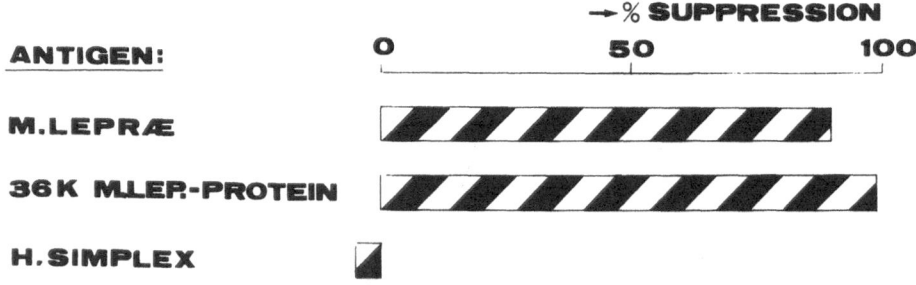

Fig. 2

Antigen specific suppression of peripheral T cell responses against a purified *M. leprae* 36K protein. The results are expressed as the percentage suppression after the addition of 3×10^4 T suppressor cells (see legend table 1). The response in the absence of T suppressor cells against the 36K protein was 12,020 cpm, against *M. leprae* 27,040 cpm, and against HSV 14,255. Responses with no antigen in the culture were 1,030 cpm in the absence and 428 cpm in the presence of the T suppressor cells. Standard deviations did not exceed 20%. The suppressor T cell line was tested in this experiment. Similar results have now been obtained with Ts clones. The tested 36K protein was purified by affinity chromatography using monoclonal antibody F47–9–1 (14,15) coupled to cyanogen bromide-activated Sepharose 4B, followed by elution with 0,1 M diethylamine pH 11,5. The protein was tested in a concentration of 5,6 μg ml^{-1}.

This may be true for the 36K protein as well. A second explanation however for the suppression of Th cell responses against the 36K *M. leprae* protein would be that that Ts cells specifically recognize (an) idiotypic determinant(s) on the 36K responsive Th cells. Whatever the mechanism of the observed suppression, it is clear that the activation of antigen specific suppressor cells places constraints on the use of such proteins for prophylactic immunization. We hope that a suppressor epitope will turn out to be the right explanation, because then the rational design of a synthetic *M. leprae* vaccine would imply the selection of helper epitopes and/or the molecular dissociation of helper from suppressor epitopes (22). If the mechanism would appear to be an anti-idiotypic one, such a vaccine strategy would not easily result in the circumvention of *M. leprae* reactive suppression in susceptible individuals.

In order to obtain more insight into the specificity and mechanism of the suppression mediated by these Ts clones, we isolated CD4 positive clones from the same patient that proliferated to *M. leprae* by cloning the cells relatively early (96 hours) after a single exposure to *M. leprae*. This procedure was followed because helper T cell growth was reported to preceed that of suppressor T cells in time (23). The thus isolated supposedly Th clones responded to *M. leprae* specific or crossreactive determinants, like was observed for tuberculoid patients and healthy contacts (16,24) and were HLA-DR or -DP restricted in their response. As shown in Table 2, Ts clones could suppress both *M. leprae* specific and

Table 2

Ts clones suppress the *M Leprae* response of some but not all *M. Leprae* reactive Th clones of the same patient.

Proliferative Th clone:	2F9	2B2	2F6
Proliferation to *M. leprae*:	+	+	+
Proliferation to other mycobacteria:	−	±	+
Ts clone added	percentage suppression		
1G2	41[1]	47	63
1D11	55	52	62
1E9	5	−1	30
1D10	−51	−13	4

Results are expressed as the percentage suppression (see legend table 1). *M. leprae* specific (2F9), partly crossreactive (2B2) or completely crossreactive (2F6) Th clones of the same patient were induced to proliferate by autologous irradiated APC and *M. leprae* antigen as described recently (16, 26). Briefly, 10^4 TLC cells were cocultured with 5 x 10^4 APC (40 Gy irradiated) and Dharmendra lepromin (1:80) for 72 hrs., after which ^{3}H-TdR was added as described in the legend of fig. 1. The mean cpm of the Th clones in the absence of suppressor T cells were 36,780 for 2 F9, 8,252 for 2B2 and 8,694 for 2F6. At the start of the culture either no or 3 x 10^4 suppressor cells were added. Background proliferation in cultures containing Th and Ts cells without antigen was always less than 440 cpm. The percentage of suppression was calculated as described in the legend of fig. 1. Standard deviations did not exceed 20%.

crossreactive Th clones in a number of cases (1G2,1D11). Other Ts clones appeared to suppress only some (1E9) or no (1D10) Th clones, although suppressing the *M. leprae* response of PBMNC. Apart from providing a (negative) control for the specific suppression on Th clones, the latter observation may either indicate that in order to complete and/or amplify the suppressor circuit, cells other than the Ts clones have to be recruited. Alternatively, the Ts clones may be anti-idiotypic and would not suppress Th clones (2F9,2B2) which carry another idiotypic determinant than that seen by the Ts cell. However, probably the most important aspect of the data presented in this table is the fact that the same Ts clones which suppressed Th responses to crossreactive mycobacterial antigens (Ts clones 1G2 and 1D11, see also table 1) are also able to suppress a Th clone directed against an *M. leprae* specific epitope. This might indicate that crossreactive Ts clones as described in this paper although not *M. leprae* specific, could play an essential role in the *M. leprae* specific unresponsiveness observed in lepromatous leprosy. It is interesting that in several instances a marked depression of *M. tuberculosis* and BCG responses has been noted in lepromatous leprosy patients (e.g. 25,26). In the light of our findings this may be explained at least in part by *M. leprae* induced crossreactive Ts cells. We deliberately selected a borderline lepromatous leprosy patient, which was not unresponsive to *M. leprae* in order to be able to generate both Th and Ts clones. Therefore we have to be cautious in generalizing this observation because it is generally assumed that lepromatous leprosy patients are nonresponsive to *M. leprae* but remain good responders towards other mycobacteria (reviewed in 1,5). Interestingly, it has recently been suggested that such patients – in contrast to tuberculoid patients and healthy contacts – do not respond to crossreactive or common antigens of other mycobacteria, but rather to the species specific antigens except of course the *M. leprae* specific ones (25,27,28; Rook, G.A.W., submitted for publication). The question then arises why the *M. leprae* induced crossreactive Ts cells could not also suppress Th responses against the species specific antigens of other mycobacteria than *M. leprae*. Extending the antigen bridging model (ref. 20,21), we propose that these Ts cells might only suppress Th cells when both the suppressor epitope (i.e. the crossreactive *M. leprae* suppressor epitope) and the helper epitope to which the *M. leprae* reactive Th cells were induced originally (i.e. either a *M. leprae* specific or a crossreactive helper epitope) are expressed by the same molecule. This prerequisite is not met in the case of Th responses against the species specific helper epitopes of other mycobacteria than *M. leprae*: since these helper epitopes by definition are not situated on molecules shared with *M. leprae*, Th responses against these non-*M. leprae* epitopes can evade suppression by crossreactive Ts cells irrespective of the presence of a crossreactive suppressor epitope on that same molecule. Qualitative and quantitative differences in the sensitization towards those species specific helper epitopes in lepromatous leprosy patients might thus account for at least part of the heterogeneity observed in responsiveness against other mycobacteria in lepromatous leprosy.

Since the observed suppression of peripheral Th cell responses and Th clones might be explained by cytotoxicity against either responding antigen specific Th cells or APC, we investigated whether peripheral T cells activated by *M. leprae* or HSV, or autologous EBV-BC, pulsed or unpulsed with *M. leprae*, or *M. leprae* reactive Th clones could be lysed by suppressor cells. However, no specific lysis of these targets by the suppressor T cell line and Ts clones was observed, whereas a control cytotoxic T cell line specific for HLA-A2 strongly lysed all targets tested. Therefore these results excluded cytotoxicity as a possible mechanism of suppression.

Finally, we were interested to know whether these Ts clones were HLA-restricted or not and if so by which HLA molecules and epitopes. Modlin *et al.* (29) have recently claimed that suppressor T cells from the skin lesions of lepromatous leprosy patients may be restricted by HLA-DR. Our own preliminary data obtained with both panel and family studies in which the Ts cells were mixed with allogeneic Th cells have indeed also shown evidence for some kind of restriction. However, this was not simply associated with HLA-class I, -DR or -DQ alleles. Thus far, we have been unable to abolish the suppression with HLA-class I or HLA-DQ specific monoclonal antibodies, but HLA-DR antibodies could do so in certain Th-Ts cell combinations. Thus, although HLA-DR might be involved, the genetic restriction of Ts cells seems to be more complex than that of Th cells.

The lines and clones described in this paper can be made available to interested colleagues. We would like to thank Prof. dr. J.J. van Rood for his support for this project; dr. R.C. Good for providing us with *M. leprae* antigen; Prof. dr. D.L. Leiker for his help and continuous cooperation; the patients for donating blood; Earl Johanns and John Haanen for technical assistance; Fons UytdeHaag for supplying HSV antigens; Madeleine de Wit for isolating the 36K protein; Arend Kolk for monoclonal antibodies; Jos Pool for his assistance in the CML test and in preparing serum pools, Annemarie Termijtelen for helpful discussions and Ellen van der Willik for preparing of the manuscript. This study was supported in part by the Foundation for Medical Research (FUNGO grant 900–509–099), the Immunology of Leprosy (IMMLEP) component of the UNDP/WORLD Bank/WHO Special Programme for Research and Training in Tropical Diseases, the Netherlands Leprosy Relief Association (NSL), and the J.A. Cohen Institute for Radiopathology and Radiation Protection (IRS).

References

1. Bloom, B.R. & Godal, T. Rev. Infect. Dis. 5,765-780 (1983).
2. Rees, R.J.W. Nature 211,576 (1966).
3. Patel, P.J. & Lefford, M.J. Infect. Immun. 19,87-93 (1978).
4. Lowe, C., Brett, S.J. & Rees, R.J.W. Clin. exp. Immun. 61, 336-342 (1985).
5. Bloom, B.R. & Mehra, V. Immun. Rev. 80,5-28 (1984).
6. Mehra, V., Mason, L.H., Fields, J.P. & Bloom, B.R. J. Immun. 123, 1813-1817 (1979).
7. Mehra, V., Brennan, P.J., Rada, E., Convit, J. & Bloom, B.R. Nature 308,194-196 (1984).
8. Nath, I., van Rood, J.J., Mehra, N.K. & Vaidya, M.C. Clin. exp. Immun. 42,203-210 (1980).
9. Sathish, M., Bhutani, L.K., Sharma, A.K. & Nath. I. Infect. Immun. 42, 890-899 (1983).
10. Salgame, P.R., Mahadevan, P.R. & Antia, N.H. Infect. Immun. 40, 1119-1126 (1983)
11. Blue, M.L., Daley, J.F., Levine, H. & Schlossman, S.F. J. Immun. 134, 2281-2286 (1985).
12. Farcet, J.P., Gourdin, M.F., Calvo, C., Oudrhiri, N., Divine, M., Bouguet, J., Fradelizzi, D., Senik, A & Reyes, F., Eur. J. Immun. 15,1067-1073 (1985).
13. Young, R.A., Mehra, V., Sweetser, D., Buchanan, T.M., Clark-Curtiss, J., Davis, R.W. & Bloom, B.R. Nature 316,450-452 (1985).
14. Klatser, P.R., de Wit, M.Y.L. & Kolk, A.H.J. Clin. exp. Immun. 62,468-473 (1985).
15. Engers, H.D., Abe, M., Bloom, B.R., Mehra, V., Britton, W., Buchanan, T.M., Khanolkar, S.K., Young, D.B., Closs, O., Gillis, T., Harboe, M., Ivanyi, J., Kolk, A.H.J. & Shepard, C.C. Infect. Immun. 48, 603-605 (1985).
16. Ottenhoff, T.H.M., Klatser, P.R., Ivanyi, J., Elferink, D.G., de Wit, M.Y.L. & de Vries, R.R.P. Nature 319,66-68 (1986).
17. Wicker, L.S., Katz, M., Sercarz, E. & Miller, A. Eur. J. Immun. 14,442-447 (1984).
18. Goodman, J.W. & Sercarz, E. Ann. Rev. Immun. 1, 465-498 (1983).
19. Lehner, T., Mehlert, A., Avery, J., Jones, T. & Caldwell, J. J. Immun. 135,1437-1442 (1985).
20. Oki, A. & Sercarz, E. J. Exp. Med. 161, 897-911 (1985).
21. Krzych, U., Fowler, A.V. & Sercarz, E. J. Exp. Med. 162, 311-323 (1985).
22. Mitchison, N.A. Nature 308, 112-113 (1984).
23. Bensussan, A., Acuto, O., Hussey, R.E., Milanese, C. & Reinherz, E.L. Nature 311,565-567 (1984).
24. Mustafa, A.S., Gill, H.K., Nerland, A., Britton, W.J., Mehra, V., Bloom, B.R., Young, R.A. & Godal, T. Nature 319, 63-66 (1986).
25. Reitan, L.J., Closs, O. & Belehu, A. Int. J. Lepr. 50, 455-467 (1982).
26. Godal, T., Myklestad, B., Samuel, D.R. & Myrvang, B. Clin. exp. Immun. 9, 825-831 (1971).
27. Smelt, A.H.M., Rees, R.J.W. & Liew, F.Y. Clin. exp. Immun. 44, 507-511 (1981).
28. Stanford, J.L., Nye, P.M., Rook, G.A.W., Samuel, N.M. & Fairbank, A.A. Lepr. Rev. 52, 321-327 (1981).
29. Modlin, R.L., Kato, H., Mehra, V., Nelson, E., Xue-dong, F., Rea, T.H., Pattengale, P.K. & Bloom, B.R. Nature 322, 459-461 (1986) .
30. Ottenhoff, T.H.M., Elferink, B.G., Hermans, J. & de Vries, R.R.P. Human Immun. 13,105-116 (1985).
31. Elferink, B.G., Ottenhoff, T.H.M. & de Vries, R.R.P. Scand. J. Immun. 22,585-589 (1985).
32. Haanen, J.B.A.G., Ottenhoff, T.H.M., Voordouw, A., Elferink, B.G., Klatser, P.R., Spits, H. & de Vries, R.R.P. Scand. J. Immun. 23, 101-108 (1986).

CHAPTER 6

MOLECULAR LOCALIZATION AND POLYMORPHISM OF HLA CLASS II RESTRICTION DETERMINANTS DEFINED BY *MYCOBACTERIUM LEPRAE* REACTIVE HELPER T CELL CLONES FROM LEPROSY PATIENTS*.

Introduction

The activation of helper T lymphocytes requires the recognition of foreign antigen in association with a self HLA class II molecule. This phenomenon is known as HLA class II restriction (1). The polymorphic class II epitopes that are corecognized by helper T cells are functionally defined as restriction determinants (RDs) (2). There are three groups of HLA class II molecules: DP, DQ and DR (3). These molecules are expressed as heterodimeric glycoproteins on the cell surface of immunocompetent cells and are composed of a heavy (α) and a light (β) chain (3). The DP and DQ regions each contain 2 α and 2 β genes whereas the DR region is known to encode 1 α and 3 β (β_1,β_2,β_3) genes (3). It has been reported that RDs for helper T cells are carried by each group of class II products, namely D/DR, DP and DQ (for references see 1,2,4). However, the exact molecules carrying these RDs as well as the epitopes involved have remained poorly characterized.

The major histocompatibility class II molecules have been defined as the products of class II immune response (Ir) genes in experimental animals (5). Such Ir genes determine the ability of an individual to generate T cell dependent immune responses against specific antigens (5). The polymorphism of these class II Ir genes results in genetically controlled differences in such T cell dependent immune responses. An important human example of class II Ir genes may be provided by leprosy, a chronic infectious disease which is caused by *Mycobacterium leprae* (6). HLA class II linked genes are known to control the type of leprosy which develops upon infection (reviewed in 7,8) as well as the cell mediated immunereactivity against *M. leprae* and related mycobacteria as measured by skin testing (7,8; chapter 7). Since both leprosy type and skin test responsiveness strongly correlate with *M. leprae* specific helper T cell reactivity, HLA class II Ir genes may regulate these helper T cell responses against *M. leprae* antigens. If so, the mechanism of such HLA class II Ir genes might be the differential presentation of *M. leprae* antigens to helper T cells by HLA class II RDs.

*Tom H.M. Ottenhoff, Saskia Neuteboom, Diënne G. Elferink, & René R.P. de Vries. J. Exp. Med., accepted for publication with minor modifications.

In this study we have systematically explored the nature of the RDs for *M. leprae* by presenting *M. leprae* antigens to T cell clones (TLC) from leprosy patients. The antigen specificity of several of these TLC has been reported recently (9, 10, 11). The molecular localization of the RDs was determined by inhibition studies with HLA class II specific monoclonal antibodies whereas the polymorphism of the RDs was analyzed by the presentation capacity of large panels of fully class II typed allogeneic antigen presenting cells (APC). The results show that the majority of the RDs for *M. leprae* resides on DR and not on DP or DQ molecules. Since DR molecules have a much higher expression than DP and DQ molecules, this result suggests that quantitative differences in the expression of class II molecules correlate with their function in the immune response. The same explanation holds true for the observation that RDs on DR molecules coded by a DR4Dw13 haplotype were located only on a subgroup of DR molecules with the highest expression. Evidence will be presented that RDs on DR molecules may be expressed as unique conformational epitopes.

Materials and methods

Cells

PBMNC (peripheral blood mononuclear cells) were isolated from heparinized venous blood from three leprosy patients (BC; R; SC) by Ficoll-Isopaque density centrifugation (specific gravity 1.077 g/ml), washed three times in Hanks' balanced salt solution (Gibco, Scotland) and resuspended in Iscove's Modified Dulbecco's Medium (IMDM) (Gibco) supplemented with streptomycin (100 μg/ml), penicillin (100 U/ml) (both Flow Laboratories, Scotland) and 10% pooled human AB serum (HS). Epstein-Barr virus transformed B cells (EBV-BC) were generated from 5 x 10^6 autologous PBMNC. Cells were frozen in 1 ml ampoulles (Nunc, Denmark) containing 1-5 x 10^6 cells, 70% RPMI 1640 (Gibco), 20% screened pooled human AB plasma and 10% dimethylsulfoxide and stored at -196°C.

Antigen

M. leprae antigen (Dharmendra) was kindly provided by Dr. R.C. Good (Centre for Infectious Diseases, Centers for Disease Control, Atlanta, U.S.A.). The preparation consisted of bacilli which had been isolated from human lepromas.

Antigen reactivation and cloning of M. leprae reactive T lymphoblasts

This was performed as described recently (10). In brief, five times 10^6 PBMNC of two tuberculoid patients (BC and R) and one borderline lepromatous leprosy patient (SC) were restimulated *in vitro* with *M. leprae* in IMDM supplemented with 10% HS. The cultures were incubated for 5 days in 24 well tissue culture trays (Falcon 3047; Becton and Dickinson, California, USA) at 37°C in a fully humidified 5% CO_2-air mixture. Enrichment for T cell blasts was obtained either by Percoll (Pharmacia, Sweden) density centrifugation or by extending the cultures for another 3-10 days in the presence of 10% interleukin-2 containing medium (IL-2; Lymfocult-T, Biotest, FRG). After the isolation of the blasts, a cell suspension was made containing 5 blasts ml^{-1} in a mixture consisting of (i) PBMNC from 3-4 random donors (10^6 c ml^{-1}, 30 Gy irradiated), (ii) autologous EBV-BC (10^5 c ml^{-1}, 50 Gy irradiated), and (iii) an optimal concentration of *M. leprae* antigen, all in IMDM supplemented with 10% HS. This suspension was plated in 96-well flat bottomed microtitre plates (Falcon 3072, Bect. Dick.) (0.1 ml per well, i.e. 0,5 T lymphoblast per well) and incubated as described above. Growing cultures were transferred to 24 well tissue culture trays (Falcon 3047, Bect. Dick.) and restimulated with 1 ml per well of the cell/antigen mixture described above. Three to four days later IL-2 (10%) was added. After an additional 4-7 days, the cultures were restimulated again until a minimum of $2x10^6$ cells per culture was obtained. The cells were then frozen or expanded further by restimulation as described above for 4 days except that Leuko Agglutinine (Pharmacia) was added to the cell antigen mixture (final concentration: 1 μg ml^{-1}) in order to increase the yield of cells. This was followed by culturing for 3-5 days in the presence of IL-2.

Proliferative assays

$1x10^4$ TLC (0.05 ml) and $5x10^4$ irradiated (40 Gy) autologous or allogeneic PBMNC as APC (0.05 ml) were cultured in IMDM with 10% HS with 0.1 ml of *M. leprae* antigen (1/120 dilution) in 96 well flat bottomed microtitre plates (Greiner, FRG). PHA (Wellcome Diagnostics, England; 4 μg ml^{-1}) and plain IMDM were used as controls. The cultures were set up in duplicate or triplicate and incubated as described above for 72 hours. Eighteen hours before termination, 1.0 μCi of ^{3}H-thymidine (specific activity 5.0 Ci $mmol^{-1}$, Radiochemical Centre, England) in 0.05 ml RPMI 1640 was added. The samples were harvested on glass-fibre filters using a semi-automatic sample harvester. ^{3}H-thymidine incorporation was assessed by counting in a liquid scintillation counter (Searle, Nuclear, Chicago, USA). All cells had been typed for HLA-A, B, C, DR, (including DRw52 and DRw53), DQ and DP as mentioned in ref. 2. In addition, a number of cells were also typed for the cellularly defined HLA-D determinants, using homozygous typing cells and primed lymphocyte typing reagents as described in ref. 12, 13.

Monoclonal antibodies (moabs)

The monoclonal antibodies used in this study were provided generously by F. Koning unless mentioned otherwise and were PdV5.2 (anti class II mono-morphic, recognizing DR, DP and approximately half of the DQ molecules; IgG1), B9.12.1 (anti class I monomorphic; IgG2a; gift of B. Malissen), B8.11.2 (anti DR monomorphic; IgG2b; gift of B. Malissen), 7.3.19.1 (anti DRw52-like, IgG2b). SPV-L3 (anti DQ monomorphic; IgG2a; gift of H. Spits), B7/21 (anti FA- or DP monomorphic, IgG; gift of F. Bach), IIB3 (anti DQw1-like; IgG2b), TA10 (anti DQw3-like; IgM; gift of H. Maeda), 109d6 (anti DRw53-like;IgG2a; gift of R. Winchester) IC2 (anti class II monomorphic; IgG2a), LD1.1 (anti DR monomorphic; IgM), Tü22 (anti DQ monomorphic; IgG2a; gift of A. Ziegler), Genox 3.53 (anti DQw1-like; IgG1; gift of J. Bodmer), OKT3 (anti CD3; purchased from Ortho Diagnostic Systems, New Jersey, U.S.A.), RIV-6 (anti CD4; IgG2a; National Institute of Public Health, Bilthoven, the Netherlands), FK18 (anti CD8; IgG3), FK24 (anti CD11; IgG1), anti Leu7 (anti human natural killer cell-like; IgM; purchased from Bect. & Dick.) and PL15 (anti DP monomorphic; gift of R. Knowles). All moabs consisted of mouse derived ascites except for Tü22 which was the supernatant of a hybridoma culture. All moabs are described in ref. 14.

Inhibition of antigen specific TLC proliferation by moabs.

Cultures were set up as described in the fourth paragraph except that the same amount of antigen was added in only 0.05 ml. At the start of the culture, 0.05 ml IMDM with moab was added. All moabs were filter-sterilized through 0.22-μm filters (Gelman, Michigan, USA) and tested in a final completely saturating concentration of 1:50-1:200 from the original ascites.

Gamma-interferon (γ-IFN) assay

Culture supernatants of antigen activated TLC as described above were measured in duplo for levels of γIFN after 90 hours by a solid phase radio-immunoassay (Centocor Malvern, USA), using two distinct anti-γIFN moabs. The first moab had been coupled to polystyrene beads, the second had been labeled with ^{125}I and was added to the first after the addition of culture supernatant and washing the beads. Unbound labeled moab was then removed by washing. Bound radioactivity was determined by gamma scintillation counting. γIFN concentrations of the measured samples were derived from a standard curve and expressed as units ml^{-1}.

Table I.

Activated *M. leprae* reactive T cell clones produce γ-interferon

		γ-IFN production (U/ml)		proliferative response (cpmx10⁻³)	
	M. leprae:	+	–	+	–
TLC					
RI 1G5		1.9	0.1	14.2	0.0
RI 1 E4		40.3	0.1	57.9	0.1
RI 2 F9		27.2	0.1	88.4	0.1
RI 3 B4		6.0	0.1	42.2	0.2
RI 1 F9		14.5	0.2	10.0	0.1
RI 3 E8		24.8	0.1	70.5	2.3
polyclonal T-LB		22.4	0.1	53.7	0.1

M. leprae antigen was presented to 6 TLC and one polyclonal T-lymphoblast (T-LB) culture of the same patient by class II compatible APC in quadruplicate. Two cultures were assayed for ^{3}H-TdR incorporation by the T cells whereas the supernatant of the two remaining cultures was tested for γIFN production (see materials and methods).

Results

Cell surface marker phenotype of and γIFN production by activated TLC.

In order to characterize the nature of the TLC obtained, we first studied the cell surface antigens expressed by these TLC. All TLC had the CD3⁺CD4⁺CD8⁻ phenotype and were strongly positive for HLA-DR. In contrast, the expression of DQ varied from negative to strongly positive (data not shown).

Helper TLC are known to produce γIFN upon antigen activation. γIFN is a major macrophage activating factor and as such an important mediator for the induction of killing of intracellular parasites such as *M. leprae* (15). The correlation between *M. leprae* induced γIFN production *in vitro* and T cell mediated immune responsiveness *in vivo* and *in vitro* has been established clearly (16). The data presented in table I show that the TLC tested (n=6) and the parental polyclonal T lymphoblast culture produce γIFN upon activation with *M. leprae*. A poor correlation was observed between proliferation and γIFN production (r=0.45).

Based upon the membrane-phenotypes, γIFN production, class II restricted proliferative responses to *M. leprae* antigens (vide infra) and the inability to suppress other helper T cell responses against *M. leprae* (11), the TLC described in this paper were defined as helper TLC.

Definition of distinct restriction determinants on DR molecules coded by a HLA-DR4/Dw13 haplotype.

Nine *M. leprae* reactive proliferative TLC of patient BC were selected at random for further studies addressing their RD repertoire. All these TLC were specific for distinct antigenic determinants expressed by *M. leprae* as had been determined previously (10; unpublished observations). The HLA class II phenotype of BC is DR3,4; Dw13; DRw52,53; DQw3; DPw1,5.

The data presented in table II demonstrate that 6 of the 9 TLC tested are activated by antigen in association with DR4 or Dw13 but not DR3 related RDs. DR4 behaves like a supertypic specificity for the cellularly defined Dw4,10,13,14 and 15 determinants (12). These 6 TLC could all be inhibited completely by the same set of HLA-DR framework (DR^+) reactive moabs, but not at all by DQ, DP or class I specific moabs. Interestingly a DRw53 specific moab (109d6) which has been reported to block completely the responses of other TLC in these highly saturating concentrations (17, 18), did not block those *M. leprae* reactive helper TLC which clearly have to recognize a determinant on a DR molecule from the DR4Dw13 haplotype. Since all these inhibition patterns were identical, only one representative example (TLC VI4F3) is shown in fig. 1. These blocking studies indicate that the RDs for these TLC have to be located on the DR^+DRw53^- molecules and not on the DR^-DRw53^+ ones, which are low in expression compared to the DR^+DRw53^- molecules (19, 20). The DR^+DRw53^- molecules carry the DR4 and the DR4 related Dw allospecificities (19-24). Biochemical studies have demonstrated the presence of only one such a DR^+DRw53^- ($\alpha\beta_1$) complex in DR4Dw13 homozygous individuals (19-24) which implies that the RDs also have to reside on that same molecule.

Five different and reproducible clusters of TLC responses were observed as evident from table II. In the case of TLC II1D4, antigen induced responses closely followed the presence of the DR4 epitope on the APC (p=0.002) irrespective of the corresponding Dw phenotype. The responses of 5 other TLC (the left 5 in table II) were closely associated with the Dw13 determinant. These latter TLC could not be activated by APC expressing the other DR4 associated Dw specificities, namely Dw4, Dw10 and Dw14. No Dw15 positive APC were tested since this specificity is only observed in Oriental populations (12). In this group of 5 TLC, 4 related but distinct Dw13 associated clusters were observed: in one cluster (VI5E7; VI4F3) TLC responsiveness followed exactly the presence of the Dw13 specificity on the APC whereas in the other three cases respectively 6 (VI5B11), 5 (II1E3) and 3 (VII1E8) of the 7 Dw13 positive APC were able to activate these TLC in the presence of optimal concentrations of *M. leprae* antigens; these latter three different clusters thus are associated with but clearly not identical to the Dw specificity.

It should be mentioned that TLC restricted either by the serologically defined DR specificities or by Dw specificities subdividing the associated DR antigen have been described also for other haplotypes, including DR4Dw14 (25) and

83

Table II

M. leprae reactive T cell clones are restricted by several restriction determinants associated with DR and/or Dw specificities coded by a DR3 and a DR4Dw13 haplotype.

	APC				TLC BC								
					VI	II	VI	VI	VI	II	II	II	II
Nr.	DR(w)	Dw¹	DQw	DPw	1E8	1E3	5B11	5E7	4F3	1D4	1E10	2F10	4A4
Aur² 3,4	52.53	13	3	1.5	34.1±0.0	11.2±2.8	30.6±0.3	29.6±1.5	19.4±5.2	11.7±0.9	5.5±0.3	5.9±1.0	26.6±5.1
2 3,4	52.53	4	2,3	4	0.4±0.0	0.1±0.0	0.1±0.0	0.2±0.1	0.2±0.1	44.6±0.0	0.1±0.3	1.2±0.5	0.1±0.0
3 3,4	52.53	4	2,3	nt	0.3±0.2	0.1±0.0	0.1±0.0	0.1±0.0	0.1±0.0	13.2±1.3	3.8±0.3	13.4±5.9	25.6±1.8
4 3,4	52.53	4	2,3	2,4	1.1±0.2	0.3±0.0	0.1±0.1	0.3±0.0	0.8±0.0	45.9±0.9	0.1±0.0	2.7±0.3	0.1±0.0
5 3,11	52		2,3	1	0.2±0.0	0.2±0.0	0.1±0.0	0.1±0.1	0.2±0.1	0.1±0.0	0.2±0.0	2.7±1.3	29.2±0.6
6 3	52		2	nt	0.2±0.0	0.1±0.0	0.1±0.0	0.3±0.1	0.3±0.1	0.2±0.0	6.8±0.3	23.8±1.2	8.6±4.1
7 3,3	52		2	4	0.3±0.0	nt	nt	0.1±0.0	0.1±0.0	nt	0.1±0.0	nt	nt
8 2,3	52		1,2	5	0.1±0.0	0.2±0.0	0.1±0.0	0.1±0.0	0.2±0.1	0.2±0.0	0.1±0.0	0.3±0.2	0.1±0.1
9 2,3	52		2	nt	0.2±0.1	0.2±0.1	0.1±0.0	0.2±0.1	0.3±0.1	nt	0.1±0.0	nt	nt
10 2,4	53	13	2,3	nt	17.1±0.9	16.5±0.7	21.1±0.4	43.0±0.4	35.4±2.1	19.7±0.2	0.3±0.1	0.4±0.2	24.6±0.2
11 4,7	53	nt	2,3	nt	0.2±0.0	0.1±0.0	0.2±0.0	32.1±1.9	46.0±3.2	63.7±1.9	0.1±0.0	0.7±0.2	0.3±0.1
12 4,13	52.53	13	1,3	nt	0.7±0.1	0.3±0.0	7.3±1.3	32.3±3.2	33.8±0.3	6.5±1.6	0.1±0.0	0.7±0.3	0.2±0.0
13 4,12	52.53	13	3	4,5	51.8±0.0	30.8±0.6	27.1±2.7	39.0±0.0	54.5±1.6	49.6±2.0	0.1±0.0	0.3±0.1	0.2±0.1
14 4	53	13	3	nt	26.3±0.5	9.5±2.5	43.8±0.9	29.5±1.5	17.2±0.2	nt	nt	nt	nt
15 4,8	52.53	13	3	nt	0.1±0.1	3.4±0.6	14.3±1.7	79.9±0.0	31.6±0.9	nt	nt	nt	nt
16 4	53	4,13	3	nt	0.9±0.3	3.7±2.6	1.0±0.6	73.3±0.7	26.5±5.6	nt	nt	nt	nt
17 4,13	52.53	13	1,3	nt	0.7±0.0	0.5±0.3	8.6±2.1	61.1±3.1	21.0±3.1	nt	nt	nt	nt

Table II

M. leprae reactive T cell clones are restricted by several restriction determinants associated with DR and/or Dw specificities coded by a DR3 and a DR4Dw13 haplotype.

| | APC | | | | TLC BC | | | | | | | | |
| | | | | | VI | II | VI | VI | VI | II | II | II | II |
Nr.	DR(w)	Dw[1]	DQw	DPw	1E8	1E3	5B11	5E7	4F3	1D4	1E10	2F10	4A4
18	4,13	4	1,3	nt	0.2±0.0	0.4±0.3	0.2±0.0	0.2±0.1	0.4±0.2	nt	nt	nt	nt
19	4,4	4	3	2	0.3±0.1	nt	nt	0.3±0.0	0.3±0.1	nt	nt	nt	nt
20	4,13	4	1,3	2.5	0.3±0.1	0.1±0.0	0.1±0.0	1.3±0.0	0.1±0.0	nt	0.1±0.0	0.9±0.1	0.1±0.0
21	2,4	4	1,3	nt	0.3±0.0	0.2±0.0	0.3±0.0	0.2±0.1	0.7±0.1	nt	nt	nt	nt
22	4,8	non-13 non-4	3	4	0.3±0.1	0.1±0.0	nt	0.9±0.4	0.2±0.1	nt	0.1±0.0	0.1±0.0	0.1±0.0
23	4,11	14	3	4	nt	0.1±0.0	nt	2.3±0.3	0.1±0.0	42.6±1.7	0.1±0.0	0.1±0.0	0.1±0.0
24	2,4	14	1,3	nt	0.4±0.1	0.3±0.0	0.2±0.0	0.4±0.1	1.4±1.0	nt	nt	nt	nt
25	4,12	10	3	4	0.7±0.3	0.1±0.0	0.2±0.1	0.1±0.0	0.1±0.0	11.0±0.6	0.1±0.0	0.1±0.0	0.5±0.5
26	2,9		1,3	3	0.1±0.0	0.1±0.0	0.1±0.0	0.1±0.0	0.1±0.0	0.1±0.1	0.1±0.0	0.1±0.1	0.1±0.0
27	1,7		1,2	4	0.3±0.0	0.8±0.7	0.2±0.0	0.1±0.0	0.3±0.0	nt	0.1±0.0	8.5±0.3	nt
28	11,11		3	2	0.3±0.0	0.3±0.1	0.2±0.1	0.2±0.1	0.4±0.1	nt	nt	nt	nt
29	-	-	-	-	0.1±0.0	0.1±0.0	0.1±0.0	0.1±0.0	0.1±0.0	0.1±0.0	0.1±0.0	0.1±0.0	0.1±0.0

Notes

M. leprae antigen was presented to several TLC derived from patient BC by a panel of allogeneic APC. The HLA class II phenotypes of the APC donors are shown. Results are expressed as cpm x 10^{-3} ± S.D. of antigen stimulated cultures. Background proliferation was 0.5 ± 0.3 x 10^3 cpm. Cultures were regarded positive when the observed cpm exceeded both 2,000 cpm and 15% of the cpm observed in case of autologous APC.

1. Only HLA-DR4 associated Dw specificities are indicated, i.e. HLA-Dw 4, 10, 13 and 14.
2. Autologous APC and class II phenotype.
3. n.t.=not tested.
4. background proliferation in the absence of antigen: 3.9±1.9

DR2Dw12 (26). However, the RDs described in these and other studies correlated with the known Dw types and did not detect an additional Dw related RD heterogeneity as shown in the present study.

In conclusion, our results indicate that in the DR4Dw13 haplotype both the serologically defined DR4 and the cellularly defined Dw13 allospecificity may be closely related to if not identical with RDs for *M. leprae*. In addition, five TLC define four Dw13 related clusters, most probably representing four distinct Dw13 associated RDs. All RDs in this haplotype were situated on the DR^+DRw53^- ($\alpha\beta_1$) molecule and not on the DR^-DRw53^+ ($\alpha\beta_3$) one which is low in expression compared to the $\alpha\beta_1$ molecule.

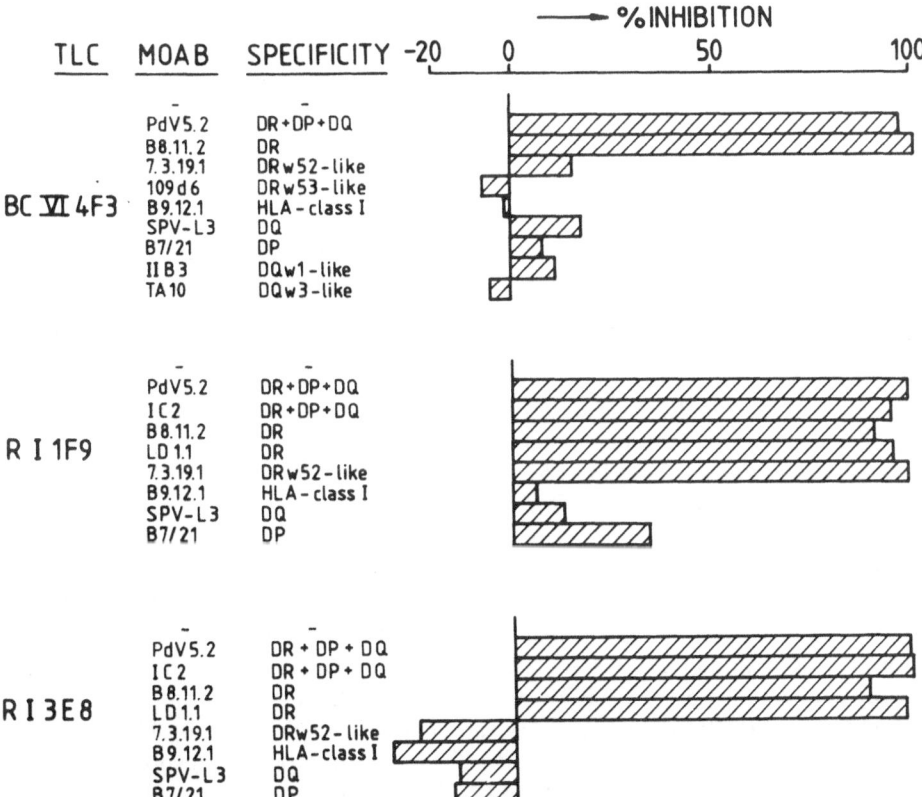

Fig. 1
Localization of restriction determinants for *M. leprae* reactive TLC on HLA-DR molecules.

Inhibition of M. leprae induced T cell responses in the presence of autologous or class II compatible APC. The results shown for TLC BCV14F3 (see table II), RI1F9 and RI3E8 (see table III) are expressed as the percentage inhibition of the TLC responses against *M. leprae* as calculated with the formula (1-cpm of TLC cultured in the presence of moab/cpm of TLC cultured in the absence of moab) x 100%. Standard deviations did not exceed 10%. Cpm in the absence of moab for VI4F3 were 31,565, for 11F9 15,075 and for I3E8 11,885.

Definition of different restriction determinants on DR molecules coded by HLA-DR3 and -DR2 haplotypes.

In order to determine the repertoire of RDs for *M. leprae* on molecules expressed by DR3; DRw52; (DQw2) haplotypes, a number of TLC derived from patient R (class II phenotype: DR2,3; DRw52; DQw1,2; DPw5) were studied as well as the three TLC of patient BC not restricted by DR4Dw13 associated determinants. So far, all TLC from patient R have been found to recognize distinct *M. leprae* protein antigens (9; W. van Schooten, T.O. *et al.*, manuscript in preparation).

As shown in table II, the three TLC of BC (II1E10, II2F10 and II4A4) recognized different determinants on several but not all DR3 positive APC. In addition, TLC II4A4 was activated by a DR3 negative APC, which was derived from a DR4Dw13 haplo-identical sib. In table III, four TLC from patient R are shown which responded to *M. leprae* plus DR3 positive APC. Four other TLC showed an identical pattern and therefore are not shown. Inhibition studies revealed that all TLC of BC and R restricted by DR3 associated determinants could be inhibited by moabs reactive with DR framework (DR$^+$) structures as well as by moab 7.3.19.1 that recognizes a DRw52-like specificity. In fig. 1 one representative example for these TLC is shown (RI1F9). No or only weak inhibition was observed in case of DP, DQ, or class I specific moabs. Using an other DR specific moab, the RDs of the TLC from patient R which in panel as well as in the mentioned inhibition studies reveal identical patterns could be subdivided on the base of differences in inhibition (data not shown here). Taken together, these results indicate that all DR3 related RDs reside on molecules which carry both DR and DRw52 like determinants.

To determine the RDs for *M. leprae* expressed by class II molecules on DR2, (DQw1) positive APC, TLC of patient R and of patient SC (class II phenotype: DR2,4; Dw13; DRw53; DQw2,3) were studied in more detail. The results are summarized in table III and IV. From table III it is evident that several TLC are restricted by DR2 associated determinants. Only four out of 14 TLC, all displaying a similar DR2 associated pattern are shown in the table. Although only one Dw12 positive APC could be tested, the TLC responses seem to be associated with the DR2 specificity rather than with the Dw2 or 12 specificities on the APC. Also the polyclonal T cell line of this patient responded equally well to Dw2$^+$Dw12$^-$ as to Dw2$^-$Dw12$^+$ APC (not shown here). The results for three TLC of patient SC which were (also) restricted by DR2 associated determinants in panel studies are summarized in table IV (II2F9, II2B2, II2F5). The antigen specificity of these TLC was described recently (11). In this case no DR2$^+$Dw2$^-$Dw12$^+$ APC were tested. Inhibition studies performed with these TLC from patient R and SC pointed out that all DR framework reactive moabs (n=4) completely inhibited the proliferation of these TLC whereas no inhibition was observed in case of moabs specific for DP, DQ, class I or DRw52. Therefore, only one representative example is shown in fig. 1 (RI3E8).

Table III
HLA-DR is associated with the main restriction determinants for *M. leprae* reactive TLC in a DR2 and a DR3 haplotype.

Nr.	APC					TLC								
	DR(w)		Dw'	DQw	DPw	12E4	11E4	11E3	11F9	12F10	12F9	13E8	12G4	13F10
Aut'	2,3	52	nt	1,2	5	44.7±2.7	45.9±4.5	22.3±2.0	21.2±2.3	27.2±0.3	54.6±2.8	38.2±1.5	15.2±3.6	37.4±0.4
2	2,2		2	1	4	0.4±0.0	0.9±1.0	0.3±0.1	0.1±0.0	41.7±1.6	74.7±11.2	39.7±4.4	33.3±0.3	0.4±0.1
3	2,2		2	1	4	0.2±0.0	0.1±0.0	0.1±0.0	0.1±0.0	31.7±1.5	57.8±1.2	70.3±2.8	25.1±4.2	0.3±0.0
4	2,2		2	1	2	0.4±0.0	0.3±0.2	0.1±0.0	nt	31.0±2.2	52.7±0.6	nt	18.3±2.0	0.3±0.2
5	2,2		2	1	2	0.5±0.3	0.1±0.0	0.3±0.2	nt	36.1±1.9	60.1±1.3	nt	21.7±2.8	nt
6	2,2		12	1	nt^b	0.8±0.4	0.3±0.0	0.3±0.2	nt	49.7±0.0	118.0±1.2	nt	4.1±0.0	0.2±0.1
7	3,3	52	3	2	2	35.3±2.1	41.9±2.9	24.2±1.7	41.4±2.5	0.1±0.0	0.2±0.0	0.2±0.0	0.1±0.0	0.7±0.2
8	3,3	52	3	2	1,4	77.3±0.7	67.2±0.7	44.1±0.4	29.5±1.4	0.2±0.0	0.5±0.1	0.2±0.0	0.8±0.6	0.2±0.1
9	3,3	52	3	2	4	45.4±3.6	48.3±1.9	28.7±2.0	nt	0.1±0.0	0.6±0.7	nt	0.7±0.6	0.2±0.0
10	3,3	52	3	2	4	7.7±1.1	8.5±3.0	2.8±1.4	nt	0.1±0.0	0.2±0.1	nt	0.2±0.0	nt
11	1,1			1	2	0.4±0.2	0.2±0.0	0.1±0.0	0.1±0.0	0.1±0.0	0.2±0.1	0.3±0.0	0.3±0.2	0.0±0.0
12	13,13	52		1	2,4	0.4±0.3	0.3±0.2	0.1±0.0	0.3±0.1	0.1±0.0	0.2±0.0	0.2±0.0	0.2±0.2	0.0±0.0
13	4,7	53		2,3	2,4	0.1±0.0	0.1±0.1	0.1±0.0	0.2±0.0	0.2±0.1	0.4±0.0	0.2±0.0	8.0±3.9	nt

Table III
HLA-DR is associated with the main restriction determinants for *M. leprae* reactive TLC in a DR2 and a DR3 haplotype.

Nr.	DR(w)		Dw'[1]	DQw	DPw	12E4	11E4	11E3	11F9	12F10	12F9	13E8	12G4	13F10
	APC					TLC								
14	4,7	53		2,3	4	2.1±1.1	1.1±1.1	nt	nt	0.1±0.1	nt	nt	22.7±5.4	nt
15	5,5	52		3	2	0.3±0.1	0.3±0.2	0.1±0.0	nt	0.1±0.0	0.2±0.0	nt	0.2±0.1	0.9±0.4
16	10,13	52		1	5	0.3±0.1	0.3±0.1	nt	nt	0.1±0.0	nt	nt	0.1±0.0	0.9±0.9
17	4,13	52,53		1,3	5	0.3±0.0	0.1±0.0	0.1±0.0	0.1±0.1	0.1±0.0	0.1±0.0	0.1±0.0	0.3±0.1	9.0±0.6[5]
18	2,3	52	nt	1,2	nt									0.1±0.0
19	2,3	52	nt	1,2	1,4									0.2±0.1
20	2,3	52	nt	1,2	3,4	nt	nt			nt	nt		nt	0.2±0.1
21	2,3	52	nt	1,2	1,4									0.8±0.9
22	2,3	52	nt	1,2	nt									0.4±0.2

Notes

HLA class II restriction of *M. leprae* activated TLC of patient R. See legend Table II.

1. Only DR2 or DR3 related HLA-Dw specificities are shown.
2. Autologous APC and class II phenotype.
3. Proliferative response in the absence of antigen: 8.6±1.7
4.   "   "   "   "   "   :21.9±7.3
5.   "   "   "   "   "   : 6.7±1.5

Antigen induced proliferative responses were negative in 3–5 after substraction of background proliferation.

6. n.t.=not tested.

Table IV
HLA-DR associated restriction of *M. leprae* reactive TLC.

Effect of sharing or mismatching of class II antigen between T cell
and APC on T cell responsiveness.

TLC[1]	HLA class II antigen analyzed	class II shared: TLC response:	yes yes	yes no	no yes	no no	p-value
SCII2B2	DR2[3]		5	0	0	18	0.00006
SCII2F5	DR2[3]		3	0	0	12	0.004
SCII2F9	DR2[3]		3	0	0	12	0.004
SCII2F6	DR2		1	4	12	6	0.176
	DR4		5	0	8	10	0.076
	DQw2		6	4	7	6	1.000
	DQw3		10	2	3	8	0.020
	DRw53		13	2	0	8	0.0002
	DPw1–7[4]						>0.30

Notes
1. *M. leprae* antigen was presented by allogeneic APC to TLC derived from leprosy patient SC. The HLA class II phenotype of this patient was DR2,4; Dw13; Drw53; DQw2,3.
2. The TLC-APC combinations in which the analyzed class II antigen was shared between TLC and APC were compared with regard to the observed TLC proliferative responses to the responses observed in the TLC-APC combinations mismatched for that class II antigen. The significance of the results are given as Fisher's exact p-values. Positive responses ranged from $1,2\pm0,2$–$40,2\pm0,4$ cpm; negative responsed ranged from $0,0\pm0,0$–$0,2\pm0,,0$ cpm.
3. These TLC were also tested for sharing DR4, DQw2, DQw3, DRw53 and DP antigens; all p-values obtained exceeded 0.25 (data not shown).
4. Since the T cell donor was not typed for DP, all known (w1–7) allospecificities were analyzed in the same way. The p-values obtained varied between 0.30 and 0.72 as summarized in the table.

Recently, evidence has been presented suggesting that the DR2 determinant is situated on DR $\alpha\beta_1$ complexes which are distinct from those carrying the Dw2/12 determinants, namely the $\alpha\beta_2$ complexes (26). Moreover, RDs for streptococcal as well as measles antigens displayed a preference for the $\alpha\beta_2$ and not the $\alpha\beta_1$ complex (26,27). Our data suggest that in contrast the *M. leprae* RDs show a preference for the $\alpha\beta_1$ complex.

In conclusion, our results suggest that also in case of the class II molecules expressed by DR2, (DQw1) haplotypes, RDs for *M. leprae* reside almost exclusively on DR molecules. It is likely that most RDs for *M. leprae* are located on the DR $\alpha\beta_1$ molecules which express the DR2 but not the Dw2 or Dw12 determinants.

New restriction determinants defined on DQ and DP molecules

TLC I3F10, shown in the uttermost right column of table III, was activated only by *M. leprae* plus autologous but not allogeneic APC (n=32, only 17 of which are shown) including cells derived from individuals originating from the same ethnic group. Inhibition studies showed that antigen induced responses were inhibited completely by a moab reactive exclusively with DQ molecules (SPV-L3; fig. 2A) and by only one of the two moabs reactive with monomorphic class II determinants. Partial inhibition was observed in case of moab Tü22 and Genox 3.53 reactive respectively with a monomorphic DQ and a DQw1 determinant. The weak inhibition observed in case of moab LD1.1 may be due to crossreactivity with DQ determinants. In conclusion, this TLC recognizes a RD on DQ molecules which is only expressed by autologous and not by 32 other allogeneic APC.

TLC II2F6, shown in table IV, recognizes *M. leprae* in association with a variety of allogeneic APC. Positive responses correlated best with the sharing of the DRw53 specificity between APC and TLC (p> 0.0002), less significantly so with DQw3 (p=0.02), and not with DR2 or DR4. Since this T cell donor had not been typed for DP, we analyzed the T cell responses against all known DP allospecifities on the APC tested, namely DPw1-7. None of the DP determinants was associated with T cell responsiveness (p> 0.30) excluding an association between the RD and one of the known DP specificities. Unexpectedly however, blocking studies revealed that the RD is situated on a DP molecule, since moab B7/21 was able to inhibit proliferation completely (fig. 2B). Moab PL15 which is also directed against DP determinants showed only marginal inhibition. Thus, the RD recognized by this TLC is situated on a DP molecule, does not correlate with currently known DP allospecificities and is frequently expressed among the population of APC tested (13/23).

Alloreactivity of class II restricted M. leprae *reactive TLC.*

Three regular class II restricted *M. leprae* reactive TLC were found to crossreact with some but not all allogeneic APC in the absence of antigen. These TLC were BCII2F10, shown in table II (APC nr. 27), RI2G4 (table III, APC nr. 13, 14) and RI3F10 (table III, APC nr. 17). One of these three TLC, namely RI2G4, was analyzed in more detail by means of panel and inhibition studies, and was found to recognize a DPw4 related allodeterminant (unpublished observations).

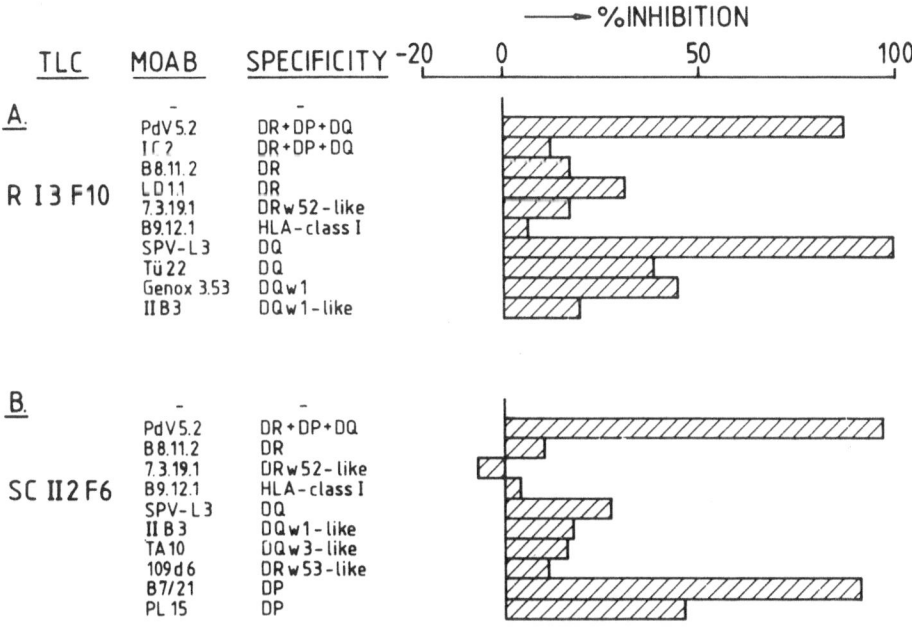

Fig. 2
Inhibition patterns of an HLA-DQ and an HLA-DP restricted *M. leprae* reactive TLC.

Inhibition of *M. leprae* induced T cell responses in the presence of autologous or class II compatible APC. The results are expressed as the percentage inhibition (see legend figure 1). Standard deviations did not exceed 10%. Cpm in the absence of moab for 13F10 were 40,545 and for II2F6 5,400.

Discussion

In this report we have defined the HLA class II molecules and characterized the polymorphic epitopes or restriction determinants (RDs) on these molecules which, in association with *Mycobacterium leprae* antigens, are recognized by cloned *M. leprae* reactive helper T lymphocytes from leprosy patients. The molecular localization of the RDs was defined by inhibition studies with HLA class II specific monoclonal antibodies whereas the polymorphism of these RDs was determined in panel studies with fully class II typed allogeneic APC. The reason why we were interested in defining these RDs is based on two facts. Firstly, polymorphic HLA class II linked Ir genes have been shown to determine T cell mediated immune responsiveness against *M. leprae* and related mycobacteria *in vivo* (reviewed in 7,8; chapter 7) as well as the type of leprosy that develops upon infection in susceptible individuals (7,8). Secondly, MHC class II molecules are involved in the restriction and regulation of antigen presentation to helper T cells and as such have been defined as the products of class II Ir gene products (ref. in 5,8). We reasoned therefore that the Ir genes that regulate the *in vivo* immune response against *M. leprae* may actually code for RDs which restrict and regulate the (*in vitro*) presentation of *M. leprae* antigens to helper T cells. The definition of such RDs is crucial for the unravelling of the mechanism of this HLA-disease association.

Our first conclusion is that the majority of the RDs for *M. leprae* is located in the polymorphic domains of HLA-DR molecules, and not on DP or DQ molecules. Thus DR molecules play a major role in the presentation of *M. leprae* antigens to T cells from leprosy patients. Since these same molecules also express the DR allospecificities that are associated with the regulation of immune responses against *M. leprae in vivo* (vide supra), it is very likely that those HLA-DR coded RDs are closely associated with if not identical to the *M. leprae* specific HLA class II Ir gene products. It has been established that the expression of DR molecules is much stronger than that of DP (14, 28, 29) and DQ (14, 29) molecules. Quantitative differences in the expression of the different class II molecules can result in significant differences in their function in immune responses as has been shown by studies in mice (30): subtle differences in the expression of I-A and I-E molecules could lead to profound alterations in immune responsiveness. Recently, we have suggested that a similar situation exists for human polyclonal T cell responses in that they are restricted preferentially by the group of DR molecules which was highest in expression on APC (31). Our findings here suggest that the quantitative differences in the expression of DR as opposed to DP and DQ are responsible for the almost exclusive localization of *M. leprae* RDs on DR molecules.

The association of RDs for other antigens than *M. leprae* with the DR allospecificities has been known for some time (e.g. 1,2). However, the precise molecular localization of such RDs has remained poorly defined in most cases.

In the case of DR molecules in DR4$^+$ cells, two types of DR molecules are expressed namely DR$^+$DRw53$^-$($\alpha\beta_1$) and DR$^-$DRw53$^+$ ($\alpha\beta_3$) molecules (19-24), the DR4 β_2 gene being a pseudogene (32). Our inhibition studies localized the *M. leprae* RDs only on the $\alpha\beta_1$ and not on the $\alpha\beta_3$ molecules. In analogy to the preferential localization of the *M. leprae* RDs on DR and not on DP or DQ molecules as a consequence of quantitative differences in the expression of DR versus DP and DQ molecules, these DR4 $\alpha\beta_1$ molecules carrying the *M. leprae* RDs have a significantly higher expression than the DR4 $\alpha\beta_3$ molecules (19,20). It is of interest to note that the DRw53$^+$ molecules are capable of presenting other antigens than *M. leprae* to helper T cells, such as mumps virus (17) and *Chlamydia trachomatis* (18).

In the case of DR molecules expressed by DR2 positive cells, qualitative rather than quantitative differences between different DR molecules may be of importance for the localization of RDs for *M. leprae*. Recently, two distinct DR2 related DR molecules were described, one probably carrying the DR2 determinant ($\alpha\beta_1$), the other one expressing the Dw2 or Dw12 specificities ($\alpha\beta_2$) (26). Both molecules were shown to be capable of stimulating allogeneic mixed lymphocyte cultures as well as presenting antigen to helper T cells. Of interest here is that in this as well as in a second study (27) the RDs for respectively streptococcal and measles virus antigens were mapped mainly to the $\alpha\beta_2$ and not to the $\alpha\beta_1$ molecules. Our results may suggest that RDs for *M. leprae* show a preference for the $\alpha\beta_1$ complex; thus the *M. leprae* RDs may be associated with DR2 rather than with the corresponding Dw specificities. In the case of DR molecules expressed by DR3 positive cells, inhibition studies demonstrated that the RDs for *M. leprae* were situated on DR molecules expressing both DR and DRw52-like determinants. These DR$^+$DRw52$^+$ molecules have been described previously and have been shown to carry RDs for *M. tuberculosis* as well (31). Recent biochemical evidence suggests that two such DR$^+$DRw52$^+$ β chains are expressed by DR3 positive cells (Bontrop, R.E.; personal communication). Because these two β chains may now be distinguished on the base of other moabs than those used in the present study, inhibition studies with these moabs will establish whether both or only one of these two β chains are involved in the expression of *M. leprae* RDs.

A second conclusion is that *M. leprae* RDs, at least in the case of DR $\alpha\beta_1$ molecules expressed by a DR4Dw13 haplotype, most probably are expressed as conformational epitopes which are specific for the DR molecules of that haplotype. As shown in table II, one *M. leprae* TLC recognized a DR4 associated RD irrespective of the Dw specificity of the APC. In contrast, 5 other TLC defined 4 distinct RDs associated only with Dw13. The DR4 as well as the Dw determinants are expressed on the $\alpha\beta_1$ molecule which also carries the *M. leprae* RDs (vide supra) whereas the DRw53 specificity is carried by the $\alpha\beta_3$ molecule (19-24).

Formally we cannot exclude that differences in antigen processing between different APC would result in the 4 different Dw13 associated clusters. One might envisage that some APC would lack the capacity to process effectively some *M. leprae* protein antigens while being capable of processing and presenting other ones. We think however that such an APC dependent highly antigen specific failure in antigen handling is a very unlikely explanation for the observed Dw13 associated heterogeneity. Moreover, such a supposition is not at all supported by other studies, notably those in which APC from non-responder animals were found to display normal antigen handling activity (e.g. 33).

Therefore we think that the 4 distinct Dw13 associated types of TLC responses in all probability represent 4 distinct RDs on the $\alpha\beta_1$ molecule. One RD is closely linked or maybe even identical to the Dw13 determinant, the other three Dw13 associated RDs define an additional hitherto unknown Dw13 related polymorphism of these DR $\alpha\beta_1$ molecules. Of interest now is that recently DR β_1 cDNA clones of the Dw4, 13 and 14 specificities have been sequenced and compared (34). The amino acid sequences derived from the nucleotide sequences are well different (at least 16 residues) from the amino acid sequence of the NH_2-terminal part of the DRw53 positive DR β_3 chain, which is identical within the DR4 and DR7 haplotypes (20,23). Therefore, these DR β_1 cDNA clones indeed may represent allelic Dw coding sequences. The comparison of these DR β_1 cDNA sequences has revealed that only very few (one to three) nucleotides differ between these allelic Dw specificities which results in amino acid substitutions located between the residues 71-86. These amino acids are part of the polymorphic first domain of the DR molecule (34), and likely to be placed on the outer face of the molecule (35). The mentioned amino acid differences may well be the only differences between the allelic Dw determinants since they are compatible with and can explain completely the recently described differences in DR β_1 isoelectric points (see 19,21,22).

The fact that only minimal alterations in the structure of class II molecules can profoundly influence their role in T cell activation (36), and even can change the Ir status of an animal, has been clearly demonstrated. A classical example has become the B6.C-H-2^{bm12} mutant mouse strain, in which as a consequence of only three amino acid substitutions in the first external domain of the I-A$_{\beta}^{bm12}$ chain (37), T cell responsiveness against the male H-Y antigen (38) and against beef insulin (39) is largely lost as compared to the strain of origin B6, H-2^b. Our results similarly demonstrate that the TLC described here most probably can distinguish precisely one (Dw14 vs. Dw13; see 34) till three (Dw4 vs. Dw13; see 34) amino acid differences between DR $\alpha\beta_1$ molecules. However, as far as we know, it has not been reported yet that a difference of only one residue (Dw14 vs. Dw13) can result in the expression of 4 – and maybe more – restriction epitopes. The fact that only 5 TLC recognize up to 4 distinct RDs may even suggest a still larger number of RDs. A first explanation for this unexpected complexity is that the mentioned amino acid differences give rise to conformational changes in the polymorphic first domain which in turn lead to the expression of multiple new (restriction) epitopes on the outer face of the molecule; such an expression of multiple new epitopes can occur either with or without physical or chemical association between DR β_1 and certain DR α chain sequences. A second explanation may be that so far undetected – presumably charge conserved – amino acid differences are present which do contribute to the formation of RDs, for instance residues in the second domain although this is more difficult to envisage. A third explanation lies in the differential binding of processed antigen to class II molecules (e.g. 40). Small differences in the nature of the antigen can profoundly influence its binding to class II molecules. Since as mentioned all *M. leprae* reactive TLC tested sofar recognize distinct *M. leprae* antigenic determinants ("epitopes"), the different processed peptides carrying these epitopes may bind to distinct class II structures ("desetopes") with their "agretopes" (41). This differential binding may then give rise to the induction of different conformational changes in the $\alpha\beta_1$ complex and may be reflected in the expression of several related but distinct RDs ("histotopes").

Whatever the mechanism leading to the expression of these RDs, in each of these three possibilities distinct conformational sites rather than linear sequences in the polymorphic β_1 domain seem to be responsible for the formation of RDs. This would imply that the sequencing of class II genes and molecules may not be able to elucidate the relationship between structure and function completely. Using recombinant DNA techniques and DNA mediated gene transfer into L cells, Lechler *et al.* (42) arrived at similar conclusions with regard to the conformational nature of RDs. They observed that separated residues in both halves of the polymorphic I-A β chain as well as in some cases also residues in the I-A α chain could contribute to the expression of RDs for a significant number of TLC, and that multiple distinct RDs were present on one I-A $\alpha\beta$ complex. Also in other studies, evidence has suggested the existence of conformational RDs (e.g. 43).

A third conclusion is that these *M. leprae* specific TLC define novel epitopes on DP and DQ molecules, which may be more relevant than those detected with alloantibodies, allospecific T cells or biochemical techniques. Although *M. leprae* reactive helper T cells are apparently mainly restricted by determinants on DR molecules, some clones do use RDs on DP and DQ molecules. Thus one TLC recognized a RD on a DP molecule not associated with a known DP allospecificity. Even more interesting was that another TLC (RI3F10) defined a RD on a DQ molecule which was only expressed by autologous APC but not by 32 allogeneic APC. The DQ region may therefore be much more polymorphic than assumed thus far. This may well be biologically quite important. In fact, the low frequency of DP and DQ restricted *M. leprae* reactive helper TLC observed by us may well be a considerable underestimate of *in vivo* situations as a consequence of an *in vitro* selection for clones restricted by class II molecules with the highest expression on the APC's used for restimulation. Moreover, not all T cells are helper T cells and maybe for suppressor T cells qualitative rather than quantitative differences in the expression of HLA class II molecules are more important.

Finally, we observed that several *M. leprae* reactive class II restricted helper TLC showed crossreactivity with a minority of allogeneic APC in the absence of antigen. Such a dual specificity has been described extensively for murine TLC, and recently also for a human TLC (44). One of the 3 TLC displaying this dual specificity (namely RI2G4) was studied in more detail, and was found to crossreact against a DPw4 like class II determinant. We could however not extend our studies of this interesting phenomenon because both the original TLC as well as subclones derived from that TLC lost their antigen specificity upon further expansion of the cultures. In our hands, this has been an exception for *M. leprae* reactive TLC. Whether this loss of antigen specificity preceded by the appearance of alloreactivity has any biological significance, and if so what, remains to be seen.

Summary

MHC class II molecules carry the restriction determinants (RDs) for antigen presentation to antigen specific helper T lymphocytes. This restriction of T cell activation endowes those molecules with a key role in the induction and regulation of antigen specific immune responses. Moreover class II molecules are the products of class II immune response (Ir) genes. The polymorphism of these Ir genes leads to genetically controlled differences in immune responsiveness between different individuals. An important human example is leprosy, in which HLA class II linked Ir genes determine the immune response against *Mycobacterium leprae*, the causative organism of the disease. Since the immune response against *M. leprae* is entirely dependent on helper T cells, the HLA class II linked Ir gene products may well regulate the immune response by controlling the presentation of *M. leprae* antigens to helper T cells. We therefore have investigated the HLA class II RD repertoire of *M. leprae* reactive helper T cell clones (TLC) by means of extensive panel and inhibition studies with fully class II typed allogeneic antigen presenting cells and well defined HLA class II specific monoclonal antibodies. The TLC studied (n= 36) proliferated specifically towards *M. leprae*, produced gamma interferon upon activation and had the $CD3^+CD4^+CD8^-$ phenotype.

The results show in the first place that the majority of the RDs for *M. leprae* resides on DR and not on DP or DQ molecules. This indicates a major role for DR molecules in the immune response to *M. leprae* and suggests that these molecules are the main products of *M. leprae* specific Ir genes. Furthermore, since the expression of DR molecules is much stronger than that of DP and DQ molecules, these findings suggest that the localization of RDs for *M. leprae* on class II molecules correlates with the quantitative expression of these molecules. The observation that the RDs on DR molecules coded by a DR4 haplotype were situated only on those DR molecules which are known to be highest in expression can be explained in the same way.

Secondly, 4 distinct RDs related with but not identical to the Dw13 allo-determinant were carried by the DR^+DRw53^- ($\alpha\beta_1$) molecules of a DR4Dw13 haplotype. Since the known amino acid residue differences between the allelic DR4 related Dw β_1 chains cannot explain the observed RD polymorphism, this observation suggests that multiple distinct conformational RDs unique for the DR4Dw13 haplotype are expressed by these molecules.

Only 2 out of 36 TLC were not restricted by DR. One of these TLC recognized a new DP determinant whereas the other TLC defined a remarkably polymorphic RD on a DQ molecule which was distinct from the known DQ related allospecificities. These TLC therefore define novel and functionally relevant polymorphisms on class II molecules. Finally, 3 of the 36 TLC reacted also with a restricted number of allogeneic APC in the absence of *M. leprae* antigen, indicating crossreactivity between self class II RD in combination with *M. leprae* antigens and allodeterminants.

Acknowledgements

We would like to thank Annemarie Termijtelen for making available her random panel for this study and for Dw typing, Nancy Reinsmoen (Minneapolis) for typing part of the DR4Dw specificities, prof. dr. D.L. Leiker (Amsterdam) for his help in obtaining blood samples from leprosy patients, dr. R.C. Good (Atlanta) for providing us with *M. leprae* antigen, Ronald Bontrop for stimulating discussions, John Haanen for technical assistance, Frits Koning, B. Malissen, H. Spits, F. Bach, H. Maeda, R. Winchester, A. Ziegler, J. Bodmer, and R. Knowles for generously supplying us with monoclonal antibodies, prof. van Rood for supporting this project and Ingrid Curiël for preparing the manuscript. This study was supported in part by the Foundation for Medical Research (FUNGO grant 900-509-099), the Immunology of Leprosy (IMMLEP) component of the UNDP/WORLD Bank/WIIO Special Programme for Research and Training in Tropical Diseases, the Netherlands Leprosy Relief Association (NSL), and the J.A. Cohen Institute for Radiopathology and Radiation Protection (IRS).

References

1. Thorsby, E. 1984. The role of HLA in T cell activation. Hum. Immunol. 9: 1.
2. Ottenhoff, T.H.M., Elferink, B.G., Hermans, J. and de Vries, R.R.P. 1985. HLA class II restriction repertoire of antigen specific T cells. I. The main restriction determinants for antigen presentation are associated with HLA-D/DR and not with DP and DQ. Hum. Immunol. 13: 105.
3. Möller, G. 1985. Molecular genetics of class I and class II MHC antigens. Immunol. Rev. 84, 85.
4. Ottenhoff, T.H.M., Elferink, B.G., Termijtelen, A., Koning, F., and de Vries, R.R.P. 1985. HLA class II restriction repertoire of antigen specific T cells. II. Evidence for a new restriction determinant associated with DRw52 and LB-Q1. Hum.Immunol. 13: 117.
5. Benacerraf, B. 1981. Role of MHC gene products in immune regulation. Science 212: 1229.
6. Bloom, B.R. and Godal, T. 1983.. Selective primary health care: strategies for control of disease in the developing world. V. Leprosy. Rev. Infect. Dis. 5: 765.
7. Van Eden, W. and de Vries, R.R.P. 1984. HLA and leprosy: a re-evaluation. Lepr. Rev. 55: 89.
8. De Vries, R.R.P., van Eden, W. and Ottenhoff, T.H.M. 1985. HLA class II immune response genes and products in leprosy. Progr. Allergy 36: 95.
9. Ottenhoff, T.H.M., Klatser, P.R., Ivanyi, J., Elferink, D.G., de Wit, M.Y.L. and de Vries, R.R.P. 1986. *Mycobacterium leprae* specific protein antigens defined by cloned human helper T cells. Nature 319: 66.
10 Haanen, J.B.A.G., Ottenhoff, T.H.M., Voordouw, A., Elferink, D.G., Klatser, P.R., Spits, H. and de Vries, R.R.P. 1986. HLA class II restricted *Mycobacterium leprae* reactive T cell clones from leprosy patients established with a minimal requirement for autologous mononuclear cells. Scand. J. Immunol. 23: 101.
11. Ottenhoff, T.H.M., Elferink, D.G., Klatser, P.R. and De Vries, R.R.P. 1986. Cloned suppressor T cells from a lepromatous leprosy patient suppress *Mycobacterium leprae* reactive helper T cells. Nature 322: 462.
12. Reinsmoen, N.L. and Bach, F.H. 1982. Five HLA-D clusters associated with HLA-DR4. Hum. Immunol. 4: 249.
13. Termijtelen, A., van Leeuwen, A. and van Rood, J.J. 1982. HLA-linked lymphocyte activating determinants. Immunol. Rev. 66: 79.
14. Koning, F. 1986. Identification and functional relevance of epitopes on human lymphocytes. Thesis, University of Leiden, 's-Gravenhage, J.H. Pasmans.
15. Nathan, C.F., Murray, H.W., Wiebl, M.E. and Rubin, B.Y. 1983. Identification of interferon-γ as the lymphokine that activates human macrophage oxidative metabolism and antimicrobial activity. J. Exp. Med. 158: 670.
16. Nogueira, N., Kaplan, G., Levy, E., Sarno, E.N., Kushner, P., Granelli-Piperno, A., Vieira, L., Colomer Gould, V., Levis, W., Steinman, R., Yip, Y.K. and Cohn, Z.A. 1983. Defective γ-interferon production in leprosy. Reversal with antigen and interleukin-2. J. Exp. Med. 158: 2165.
17. Ball, E.J. and Stastny, P. 1984. Antigen specific HLA-restricted human T cell clones. I. An MT3-like restriction determinant distinct from HLA-DR. Immunogenetics 19: 13.
18. Qvigstad, E., Gaudernack, G. and Thorsby, E. 1984. Antigen-specific T cell clones restricted by DR, DRw53 (MT), or DP (SB) class II HLA molecules. Inhibition studies with monoclonal HLA-specific antibodies. Hum. Immunol. 11: 207.
19. Bontrop, R.E., Schreuder, G.M.Th., Mikulski, E.M.A., van Miltenburg, R.T. and Giphart, M.J. 1986. Polymorphisms within the HLA-DR4 haplotypes. Various DQ subtypes detected with monoclonal antibodies. Tissue Antigens 27: 22.
20. Sorrentino, R., Lillie, J. and Strominger, J.L. 1985. Molecular characterization of MT3 antigens by two dimensional gel electrophoresis, NH_2-terminal amino acid sequence analysis, and southern blot analysis. Proc. Natl. Acad. Sci. USA 82: 3794.

21. Nepom, B.S., Nepom, G.T., Mickelson, E., Antonelli, P. and Hansen, J.A. 1983. Electrophoretic analysis of human HLA-DR antigens from HLA-DR4 homozygous cell lines: correlation between β chain diversity and HLA-D. Proc. Natl. Acad. Sci. USA 80: 6962.

22. Groner, J.P., Watson, A.J. and Bach, F.H. 1983. Dw/LD-related molecular polymorphism of DR4 β-chains. J. Exp. Med. 157: 1687.

23. Spies, T.R., Sorrentino, R., Boss, J.M., Okada, K. and Strominger, J.L. 1985. Structural organization of the DR subregion of the human major histocompatibility complex. Proc. Natl. Acad. Sci. USA 82: 5165.

24. Hurley, C.K., Giles, R., Nunez, G., DeMars, R., Nadler, L., Winchester, R., Stastny, P. and Capra, J.D., 1984. Molecular localization of human class II MT2 and MT3 determinants. J. Exp. Med. 160: 472.

25. Qvigstad, E., Thorsby, E., Reinsmoen, N.L. and Bach, F.H. 1984. Close association between the Dw14 (LD40) subtype of DR4 and a restriction element for antigen-specific T cell clones. Immunogenetics 20: 583.

26. Sone, T., Tsukamoto, K., Hirayama, K., Nishimura, Y., Takenouchi, T., Aizawa, M. & Sasazuki, T. 1985. Two distinct class II molecules encoded by the genes within the HLA-DR subregion of HLA-Dw2 and Dw12 can act as stimulating and restriction molecules. J. Immunol. 135: 1288.

27. Jacobson, S., Nepom, G.T., Richert, J.R., Biddison, W.E. and McFarland, H.F. 1985. Identification of a specific HLA-DR2 Ia molecule as a restriction element for measles virus specific HLA class II-restricted cytotoxic T cell clones. J. Exp. Med. 161: 263.

28. Sanchez-Perez, M. and Shaw, S. 1985. HLA-DP: current status. In: *Human class-II histocompatibility antigens. Theoretical and practical aspects-clinical relevance.* (Ferrone, S. *et al.* (ed)). Springer Verlag, New York. In the press.

29. Robbins, P.A., Maino, V.C., Warner, N.L. and Brodsky, F.M. 1985. Quantitation of class II histocompatibility antigens on gamma interferon activated human monocytes. Hum. Immunol. 14: 139.

30. Matis, L.A., Jones, P.P., Murphy, D.B., Hedrick, S.M., Lerner, E.A., Janeway, C.A., McNicholas, J.M. and Schwartz, R.H. 1982. Immune response gene function correlates with the expression of an Ia antigen. II. A quantitative deficiency in Ae: Ea complex expression causes a corresponding defect in antigen-presenting cell function. J. Exp. Med. 155: 508.

31. Bontrop, R.E., Ottenhoff, T.H.M., van Miltenburg, R., Elferink, B.G., de Vries, R.R.P. and Giphart, M.J. Quantitative and qualitative differences in HLA-DR molecules correlated with antigen presentation capacity. Eur. J. Immunol. 16: 133.

32. Larhammar, D., Servenius, B., Rask, L. and Peterson P.A. 1985. Characterization of an HLA-DR β pseudogene. Proc. Natl. Acad. Sci. USA 82: 1475.

33. Dos Reis, G.A. and Shevach, E.M. 1983. Antigen-presenting cells from nonresponder strain 2 guinea pigs are fully competent to present bovine insulin B chain to responder strain 13 T cells. Evidence against a determinant selection model and in favour of a clonal deletion model of immune response gene function. J. Exp. Med. 157: 1287.

34. Cairns, J.S., Curtsinger, J.M., Darl, C.A., Freeman, S., Alter, B.J. and Bach, F.H., 1985. Sequence polymorphism of HLA-DR β_1 alleles relating to T cell recognized determinants. Nature 317: 166.

35. Norcross, M.A. and Kanehisa, M. 1985. The predicted structure of the Ia β_1 domain. A hypothesis for the structural basis of major histocompatibility complex restricted T-cell recognition of antigens. Scand. J. Immunol. 21: 511.

36. Brown, M.A., Glimcher, L.A., Nielsen, E.A., Paul, W.E. and Germain, R.N. 1986. T cell recognition of Ia molecules selectively altered by a single amino acid substitution. Science 231: 255.

37. McKenzie, I.F.C., Morgan, G.M., Sandrin, M.S., Michaelides, M.M., Melvold, R.W. and Kohn, H.I. 1979. B6. C-H-2^{bm12}: a new mutation in the I region in the mouse. J. Exp. Med. 150: 1323.

38. De Waal, L.P., de Hoop, J., Stukart, M.J., Gleichmann, H., Melvold, R. and Melief, C.J.M. 1983. Nonresponsiveness to the male antigen H-Y in H-2 I-A-mutant B6. C-H-2^{bm12} is not caused by defective antigen presentation. J. Immunol. 130: 665.

39. Lin, C., Rosenthal, A.S., Passmore, H.C. and Hansen, T.H. 1981. Selective loss of antigen-specific Ir gene function in I-A mutant B6.H-2^{bm12} is an antigen presenting cell defect. Proc. Natl. Acad. Sci. USA 78: 6406.

40. Babbitt, B.P., Allen, P.M., Matsueda, G., Haber, E. and Unanue, E.R. 1985. Binding of immunogenic peptides to Ia histocompatibility molecules. Nature 317: 359.

41. Schwartz, R.H. 1985. T-lymphocyte recognition of antigen in association with gene products of the major histocompatibility complex. Ann. Rev. Immunol. 3: 237.

42. Lechler, R.I., Ronchese, F., Braunstein, N.S. and Germain, R.N. 1986. I-A-restricted T cell antigen recognition. Analysis of the roles of Aα and Aβ using DNA-mediated gene transfer. J. Exp. Med. 163: 678.

43. Lerner, E.A., Matis, L.A., Janeway, C.A., Jones, P.P., Schwartz, R.H. and Murphy, D.B. 1980. Monoclonal antibody against an Ir gene product? J. Exp. Med. 152: 1085.

44. Umetsu, D.T., Yunis, E.J., Matsui, Y., Jabara, H.H. and Geha, R.S. 1985. HLA-DR4 associated alloreactivity of an HLA-DR3 restricted human tetanus toxoid-specific T cell clone: inhibition of both reactivities by an alloantiserum. Eur. J. Immunol. 15: 356.

CHAPTER 7

HLA-DR3 MOLECULES ARE THE PRODUCTS OF AN HLA CLASS II IMMUNE REGULATOR GENE FOR *MYCOBACTERIUM LEPRAE* PREDISPOSING TO TUBERCULOID LEPROSY.*

Introduction

Antigen specific immune responses are controlled by polymorphic immune response (Ir) genes. In experimental animals, the majority of these Ir genes has been mapped to the major histocompatibility complex, the MHC (1,2). MHC class II Ir genes have been found to control immune reactivity against T cell dependent foreign antigens. The products of these MHC class II Ir genes are the MHC class II molecules (1,2). Three major mechanisms of MHC class II Ir gene controlled interindividual variability in immune responsiveness have been described: a) differences in the available or selected T cell-antigen receptor repertoire b) differences in the capacity of class II molecules to associate with antigen in order to create an immunogenic complex for T cells, and c) differences in the activation of functionally distinct T cell compartments, e.g. suppressor (Ts) versus helper (Th) cells (2,3).

It has been recognized that the HLA class II region contains similar polymorphic antigen specific Ir and Is (immune suppression) genes (e.g. 4,5,6). It is generally assumed that at least several of the known associations between HLA class II alleles and certain diseases may be a consequence of such HLA class II Ir/Is genes. The polymorphism of these Ir/Is genes and consequently their products would lead to genetically controlled interindividual variability in immune responsiveness and thus in susceptibility or resistance to disease. The unravelling of this chain of events not only is important for the theoretical understanding of the mechanisms of HLA-disease associations, but may also be practically relevant and lead to preventive and therapeutical applications.

A major obstacle for such studies so far has been that in nearly all HLA class II and disease associations, the supposed triggering antigens have remained unknown. As a direct consequence, it has not been proven whether HLA class II molecules are also the products of the HLA class II Ir and Is genes, like in experimental animals. One important example of HLA class II Ir genes is provided by leprosy, the chronic infectious disease caused by *M. leprae* (7). HLA class II linked Ir genes most probably control the type of leprosy which develops

* Tom H.M. Ottenhoff, Diënne G. Elferink, Jenny Kobesen, Derk L. Leiker, Rudy F.M. Lai A Fat and René R.P. de Vries. Submitted for publication.

102

upon infection (reviewed in 8,9) as well as the type of cell mediated immune reactivity against *M. leprae* and other mycobacteria in skin tests (6,8,9,10). Since both leprosy type and skin test responsiveness strongly correlate with helper T cell responsiveness against *M. leprae* (7), it is likely that the HLA class II linked Ir genes actually control these antigen specific T cell responses. Since HLA class II molecules are known to restrict and regulate antigen presentation to helper T cells (ref. in 10,11), one would expect that these HLA class II Ir genes code for class II molecules which are involved in the differential regulation of *M. leprae* specific helper T cell responsiveness. In this paper we present our studies carried out in a Surinam population where HLA-DR3 is associated with tuberculoid leprosy. Our results suggest that HLA-DR3 molecules are the products of a *M. leprae* specific immune regulator gene that regulates T cell responsiveness towards *M. leprae*.

Materials and methods

Individuals

Twenty-one unrelated leprosy patients and 126 healthy individuals originating from Surinam, South America, were studied, all of them being members of an ethnic group consisting of negroid individuals with a predominantly Caucasoid admixture. The patients were attending the Dermatology departments of the Academic Medical Centre in Amsterdam, the Dijkzigt Hospital in Rotterdam and the University Hospital in Paramaribo; they had been classified according to the five-group system described by Ridley and Jopling (12). The diagnosis was based on regular and careful clinical examination, review of the clinical histories, skin-slit smear bacteriology, histopathological examination of skin biopsies and lepromin skin testing. We selected 12 lepromatous (BL, LL) and 9 polar tuberculoid (TT) patients for the study because of our specific interest in the frequency of HLA-DR3 which had previously been reported to be significantly increased in TT and decreased in BL-LL patients of this ethnic group (13). All TT patients had received regular treatment and did not show active lesions. The healthy individuals originated from the same ethnic group and were bled both in Surinam and in the Netherlands.

HLA typing and statistics

Typing for the HLA class II specificities was performed with 80 platelet absorbed sera in the two colour fluorescence test as described previously (14, 15). The significance of the differences in HLA frequencies in TT, BL-LL patients and healthy individuals and the relative risks were calculated using Woolf's method as modified by Haldane (16).

Antigen-specific proliferation of PBMNC

Standard lymphocyte proliferation assays were performed as described previously (11). In brief, 10^5 PBMNC were cocultured with antigen in 0.2 ml of Iscove's modified Dulbecco's medium (IMDM) (Gibco, Scotland) supplemented with 100 μg ml^{-1} streptomycin, 100 U ml^{-1} penicillin (both Flow laboratories, Scotland) and 10% heat inactivated human AB serum (HS). The antigens tested were PPD (Statens Serum Institute, Denmark; final concentration of 10 μg ml^{-1}), Dharmendra lepromin containing *Mycobacterium leprae* bacilli (generously supplied by Dr. R.C. Good, CDC, Atlanta; 60^{-1}-240^{-1} dilution), ultrasonicates of *M. leprae, M. tuberculosis, M. vaccae, M. kansasii, M. avium, M. gastrii, M. scrofulaceum* and in some cases a panel of other mycobacteria (see ref. 17, 18)(kindly provided by P.R. Klatser, Royal Tropical Institute, the Netherlands; 20 μg ml^{-1}), tetanus toxoid (National Institute of Public Health, the Netherlands; 1.5 Lf ml^{-1}), *Candida albicans* (Hollister Stier, U.S.A.; 10^{-1} dilution), varidase (Lederle Lab., the Netherlands; 10^{-2} dilution), PHA (Wellcome Diagnostics, U.K.; 4 μg ml^{-1}) and medium as a negative control. The cultures were set up in triplicate in 96 well flat bottomed microtitre plates (Greiner, F.R.G.) incubated at 37°C in a fully humidified 5% CO_2-air mixture for 5 days. One μCi of ^{3}H-thymidine (Radiochemical Centre, U.K.) was added to each culture in 0.05 ml RPMI 1640 (Gibco). Eighteen hours later ^{3}H-thymidine incorporation was assessed by counting in a liquid scintillation counter (Searle, Illinois).

T cell lines (TCL)

Short time cultured *M. leprae* or PPD stimulated T cell lines respectively called TCL$_{lep}$ and TCL$_{ppd}$, were set up as described in ref. 11, 17. In brief, PBMNC of TT leprosy patients or healthy individuals were restimulated *in vitro* with either *M. leprae* (Dharmendra, 60^{-1} dilution) or *M. tuberculosis* (PPD, 10 μg ml^{-1}) in IMDM with 10% HS during 5 days in 24 well tissue culture trays (Falcon 3047, Becton and Dickinson, California) and then kept in culture for another 7-10 days in the presence of 10% interleukin-2 containing medium (Lymfocult-T, Biotest, FRG). The cultures were refreshed and/or expanded every 2-3 days. The cells were then tested for antigen specific proliferation (vide infra), frozen and used for experiments.

TCL proliferation assays

10^4 TCL and 5×10^4 irradiated (40 Gy) autologous or allogeneic PBMNC as APC were cultured as described above during 3 days in the presence of antigen. The cultures were set up in duplicate or triplicate and terminated as described above.

Statistical analysis

Optimal antigen specific stimulatory conditions were used to analyze the influence of the sharing or mismatching of HLA class II specificities between T cells and allogeneic APC. All TCL were heterozygous for HLA-DR. The parameter analyzed was the percentage relative antigen specific stimulation (% RSAG) (see 11), i.e. [the observed proliferation in a certain allogeneic T cell-APC combination divided by the observed proliferative response in that T cell-APC combination that showed the highest response within the same experiment] x 100%. Because T cells and APC identical for both HLA-DR specificities were not tested in all experiments, the highest responding T cell-APC combination in each experiment was selected from the T cell-APC combinations sharing 1 DR specificity (see results). This criterium was used consistently in all analyses. In only 6 out of the 407 tested T cell-APC combinations the % RSAG was found to exceed 100% (see results). The mentioned procedure allowed for pooling the results from different experiments. The % RSAG's for each of the tested TLC in nearly all cases were collected from one experiment. The significance of the differences in the distribution of the results in different groups was then tested by the nonparametric Mann-Whitney rank sum test.

Results

Association between HLA-DR3 and tuberculoid leprosy

A previous paper of our group has reported on the increased frequency of HLA-DR3 in TT patients as compared to healthy controls and especially BL-LL patients (13). During the present study, we typed another 9 TT patients, 12 BL-LL patients and 126 healthy controls from the same population. We also checked the diagnosis of the 29 TT patients from the first study. Six TT patients, 4 of which were HLA-DR3 positive, could not be traced back anymore and therefore were excluded from the present analysis. The statistical analysis performed on the pooled numbers is shown in table I. It is clear that HLA-DR3 is significantly increased in frequency in TT patients as compared to healthy controls (p=0.002) and BL-LL patients (p=0.001), confirming the previous findings (13), although the negative association between DR3 and BL-LL leprosy as compared to healthy controls lost its significance (p=0.14). The strength of the association as indicated by the relative risk is highest in TT⇔BL-LL (RR=7.00) and less pronounced in TT⇔ healthy controls (RR=3.30). DR3 was not associated with (TT+BL+LL) leprosy per se compared to healthy controls (p=0.24). In conclusion, HLA-DR3 is associated most strongly with TT in comparison to BL-LL leprosy, less strongly with TT as compared to healthy controls but not with leprosy per se. Combined with the results of previous studies (19,20, T.O. *et al.* submitted for publication) this indicates that the type of leprosy that develops

table I
HLA-DR3 is associated with polar tuberculoid leprosy in a Surinam negroid population.

Individuals	HLA		RR°	χ^2	p-value
	DR3	DRnon3			
healthy controls	49 (23%)	163 (77%)	} 3.30	9.93	0.002*
TT patients	16 (50%)	16 (50%)			
			} 7.00	10.85	0.001+
BL-LL patients	4 (11%)	31 (89%)			

Notes
* increased frequency as compared to healthy controls.
+ increased frequency as compared to BL-LL patients.
° RR: relative risk

upon infection is regulated by an HLA-DR3 associated gene predisposing to the high resistant TT and protecting against the low resistant BL-LL form of the disease.

HLA-DR3 is not associated with high responsiveness of peripheral T cells to mycobacteria per se but may be negatively associated with non- or low- responsiveness to mycobacteria
    The simplest hypothesis for such an HLA-DR3 associated immune regulator gene that predisposes to the high resistant but protects against the low resistant form of leprosy would be that DR3 is associated with T cell immune responsiveness against *M. leprae* and related antigens. Furthermore, one would expect such DR3 associated immune responses to be relatively strong.
    We therefore tested the peripheral T cells (PBMNC) of healthy individuals (n=99) for their response to six mycobacteria, including *M. leprae* and *M. tuberculosis*, and compared the height of the observed responses in DR3 positive (n=22) and DR3 negative (n=77) individuals. Part of the results are shown in figure 1. No significant differences in antigen induced responses were observed between DR3 positive and DR3 negative individuals, suggesting that − at least in these experimental conditions − DR3 is not associated with high responsiveness to *M. leprae*, *M. tuberculosis* and other mycobacteria per se.
    We then investigated whether DR3 was negatively associated with non-responsiveness against mycobacteria since (i) earlier evidence has been presented by our group showing that DR3 was remarkably decreased in frequency in non-

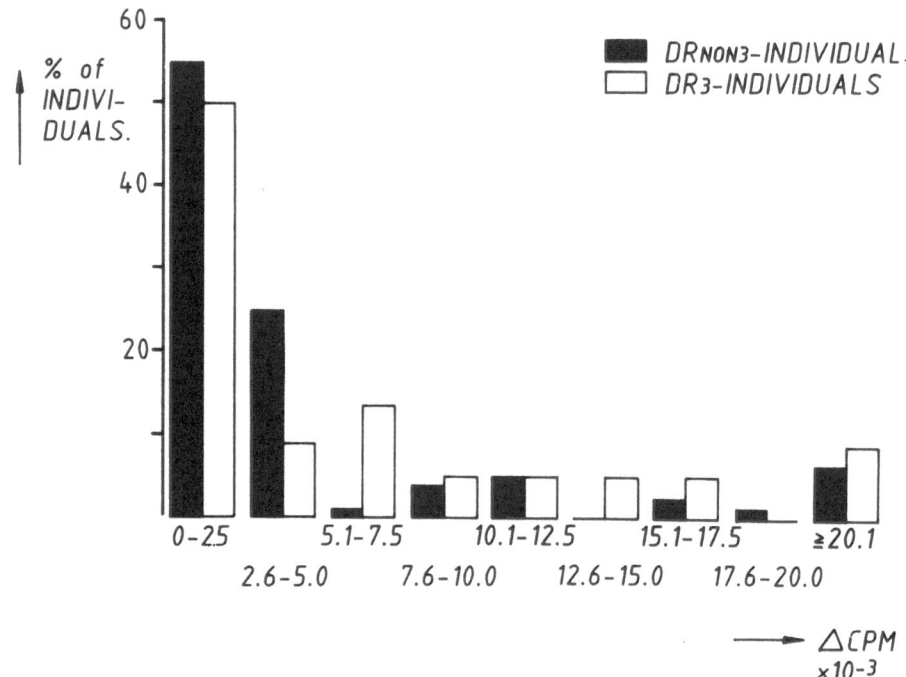

Fig. 1
Results from mycobacterial antigen induced proliferative responses of peripheral blood mononuclear cells from 99 healthy individuals. The results are expressed in Δ cpm, i.e. the observed antigen induced response minus the background proliferation for that individual. Mean background proliferation was 1,103±964 cpm (n=99). The results shown are the maximal observed responses per individual induced by one of the 6 mycobacterial antigens tested (*M. leprae*, PPD, *M. tuberculosis*, *M. avium*, *M. vaccae* and *M. scrofulaceum*). DR3 positive individuals more often show responses >5,000 cpm than DR3 negative individuals (p=0.05).

responders against mycobacterial antigens in skin testing (19) and (ii) the frequency of DR3 in (*M. leprae* low- or non-responsive) BL-LL leprosy is decreased compared to healthy controls, although not significantly, and significantly decreased compared to (*M. leprae* responder) TT leprosy (vide supra). To analyze the possible association between DR3 and low- or non- T cell responsiveness, the strongest responses of each of the 99 individuals against one of the 6 mycobacterial antigens tested were compared. These strongest responses were in all but three cases induced by *M. tuberculosis*. Nonresponders to *M. tuberculosis* never responded to one of the 5 other mycobacteria.

The mean responses in the DR3 group were 7,440 cpm, those in the DRnon3 one 5,270. Responses had been corrected for background proliferation (mean: 1,103±964 cpm) by substracting the individual backgrounds from the observed responses (Δcpm). When 5,000 cpm was taken as cut off point and thus nonresponders were defined as individuals showing antigen induced responses below 5,000 cpm, 13 of the 22 DR3 individuals (59%) were nonresponsive in contrast to 61 of the 77 Drnon3 ones (79%) (χ^2=3.67; p=0.052). When other cut off points were chosen, the observed differences did just or did not reach significance. We think we may conclude from these findings that DR3 tends to be decreased amongst *in vitro* nonresponders against mycobacterial antigens and consequently tends to be increased in the responder individuals.

Antigen specificity of M. leprae *stimulated TCL.*

Figure 2 shows that the PBMNC of a TT patient respond to different unrelated antigens (A) whereas a *M. leprae* stimulated and short time cultured TCL$_{lep}$ from the same patient only proliferated to *M. leprae* and PHA (B). Whereas this particular TCL$_{lep}$ did not respond to PPD, most TCL$_{lep}$ from other patients as well as controls did proliferate to PPD and other mycobacteria (vide infra). Thus, these TCL contain *M. leprae* specific as well as crossreactive T cells. Proliferative responses of all TCL were maximal at 72 hours. The TCL used in this study were all CD3 and HLA-DR positive and predominantly expressed the CD4 marker whereas the CD8 marker was expressed to a lower extent. No or minimal alloreactivity was seen when the TCL were cultured with allogeneic APC in the absence of antigen.

HLA-DR restriction of M. leprae *induced TCL$_{lep}$ proliferation.*

M. leprae antigen was presented to 13 *M. leprae* stimulated TCL$_{lep}$ from 13 TT patients by allogeneic APC. 197 allogeneic T cell-APC combinations were tested. The different distributions of the % RSAG in combinations with 2,1 or 0 shared DR antigens are shown in figure 3A. In the 2 DR shared T cell-APC combinations the mean % RSAG was 101.27±50.54 % (n=11), in the 1 DR shared group 42.20±32.52 % (n=127) and in the completely DR mismatched group 14.00±29.34 % (n=59). Significant differences were observed between the 2 and 1 DR shared groups (p=1.6x10^{-3}) and between the 1 and 0 DR shared groups (p=10^{-6}).

M. leprae stimulated TCL$_{lep}$ of 9 healthy controls were studied in the same manner. The results of the 148 combinations studied are shown in figure 3B. In the 2 DR shared group the mean % RSAG was 47.50±31.56% (n=10), in the 1 DR shared group 33.83±33.12% (n=95) and in the 0 DR shared one 13.84±25.13% (n=43). Significant differences were observed between the 1 and 0 DR shared groups (p=3x10^{-4}) and between the 2 and 0 DR shared groups (p=10^{-2}). The differences between the 2 versus the 1 DR shared groups did not reach significance (p=0.28) because of the unexpected absence of T cell responses in three DR identical T cell-APC combinations.

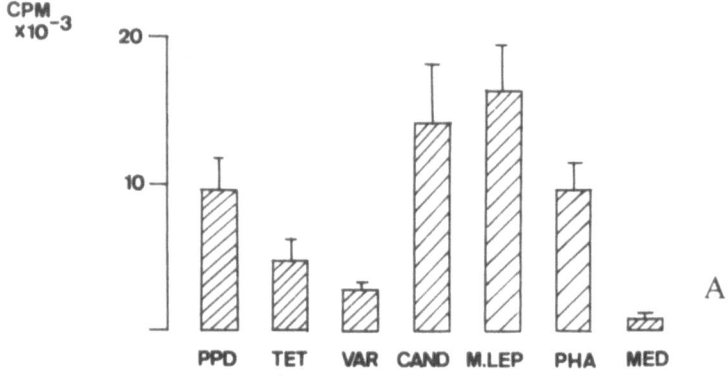

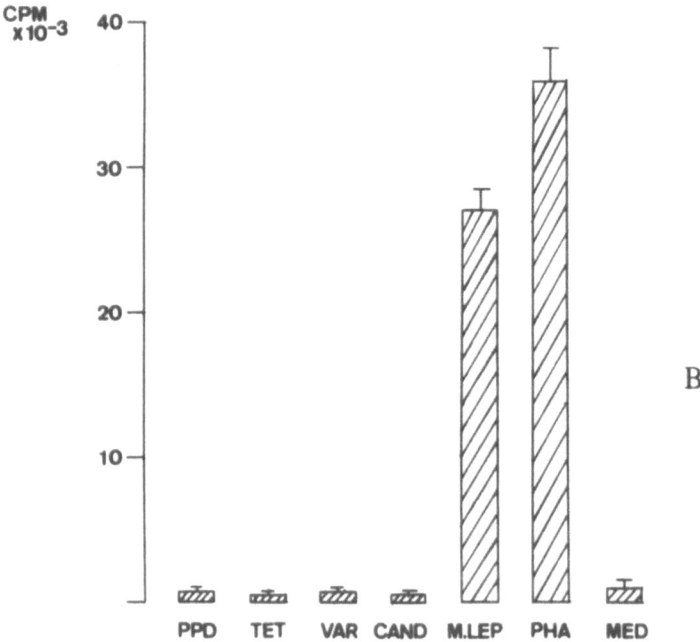

Fig. 2
Comparison of proliferative responses of PBMNC (A) with a *M. leprae* specific TCL$_{lep}$ from the same TT patient (B). The results are expressed as mean cpm ± SEM.

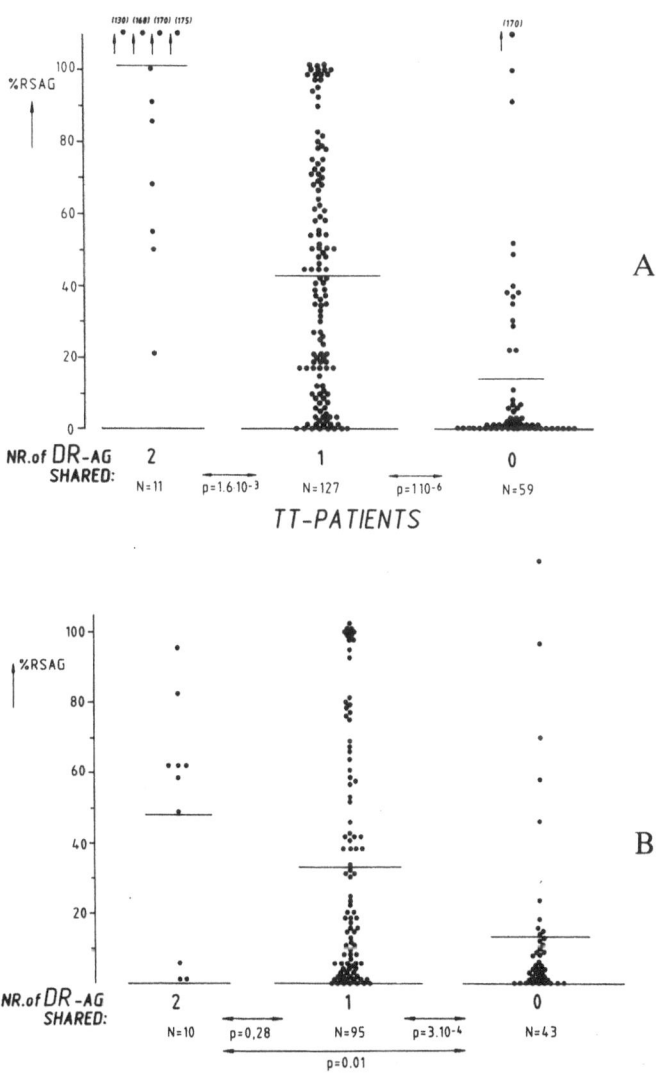

Fig. 3

A) HLA-DR restriction of *M. leprae* induced proliferation of TCL_{lep} from 13 TT patients.

B) HLA-DR restriction of *M. leprae* induced proliferation of TCL_{lep} from 9 healthy individuals.

The results are expressed in % RSAG. Mean values for the T cell-APC combination sharing respectively 2, 1 or 0 DR antigens are indicated by horizontal lines. The significance of the differences in the distribution of T cell responses between the 2, 1 and 0 DR shared groups are indicated. The 100% RSAG responses of the TCL of the patients were 6,641; 7,495; 9,107; 10,625; 10,839; 17,530; 17,917; 24,000; 32,457; 51,755; 53,807 and 59,732 cpm respectively. These of the healthy controls were 5,498; 5,894; 6,447; 6,887; 7,027; 8,500; 19,033; 40,310 and 56,023 cpm. The underlined values are those of DR3 heterozygous individuals. Standard deviations did not exceed 15%.

In conclusion, *M. leprae* specific responses of TCL_{lep} from TT patients as well as healthy controls are strongly associated with the sharing of HLA-DR antigens between T cells and APC. These results indicate that *M. leprae* specific T cell responses apparently are restricted mainly via DR. Inhibition studies with HLA class II specific monoclonal antibodies and patient derived T cell lines and clones located the restriction determinants indeed on the DR molecules (chapter 5).

M. leprae *induced T cell responses are preferentially restricted via the DRnon3 in TT patients but via DR3 in healthy individuals.*

Of the 13 TT patient derived *M. leprae* TCL_{lep}, 7 originated from DR3/non 3 heterozygous patients. To analyze the role of DR3 in the *M. leprae* induced activation of such T cells, we compared within the only 1 DR shared T cell-APC combinations (n=91) the effect of DR3 (n=51) versus DRnon3 (n=40) sharing. As shown in figure 4, a preferentially DRnon3 restricted T cell responsiveness was found (p=1.3×10^{-5}), thus confirming previous results obtained with purified peripheral T cells and allogeneic monocytes (21). No differences were observed when APC from Dutch or Surinam Caucasoid donors were used, or APC from patients or healthy individuals. Such differences were observed only for DR3 and not for the other DR antigens.

Eight *M. leprae* stimulated TCL_{lep} from healthy DR3/non3 heterozygous individuals were analyzed similarly. As shown in figure 4, in this case a preferentially DR3 restricted T cell responsiveness was found (p=6.10^{-3}). The same APC were tested as had been used for the TT patient derived TCL_{lep}. Likewise, no differences with respect to the origin of the APC were observed. The observed differences were again specific for DR3 and not observed for other DR specificities.

In conclusion, *M. leprae* reactive HLA-DR restricted T cells from DR3/non3 heterozygous TT patients are preferentially restricted by DRnon3, whereas such T cells from healthy controls are preferentially restricted by DR3.

The preferentially DRnon3 restricted responsiveness of M. leprae *stimulated* TCL_{lep} *from TT patients is specifically induced by* M. leprae *and not by* M. tuberculosis.

We next wanted to know whether patient derived TCL initially stimulated with another antigen than *M. leprae* showed a similar preferential DRnon3 restriction as the TCL_{lep}. Therefore, PPD stimulated TCL, TCL_{ppd}, were prepared from 3 TT patients. As shown in figure 5, when PPD was presented to these TLC_{ppd} via either DR3 or DRnon3 APC, the DR3 and not the DRnon3 was now associated preferentially with T cell responsiveness. (DR3 shared versus DRnon3 shared combinations: p=0.015). Mean responses in these two groups were $64.94 \pm 25.81\%$ (n=16) and $42.11 \pm 23.11\%$ (n=18). Thus, the induction of

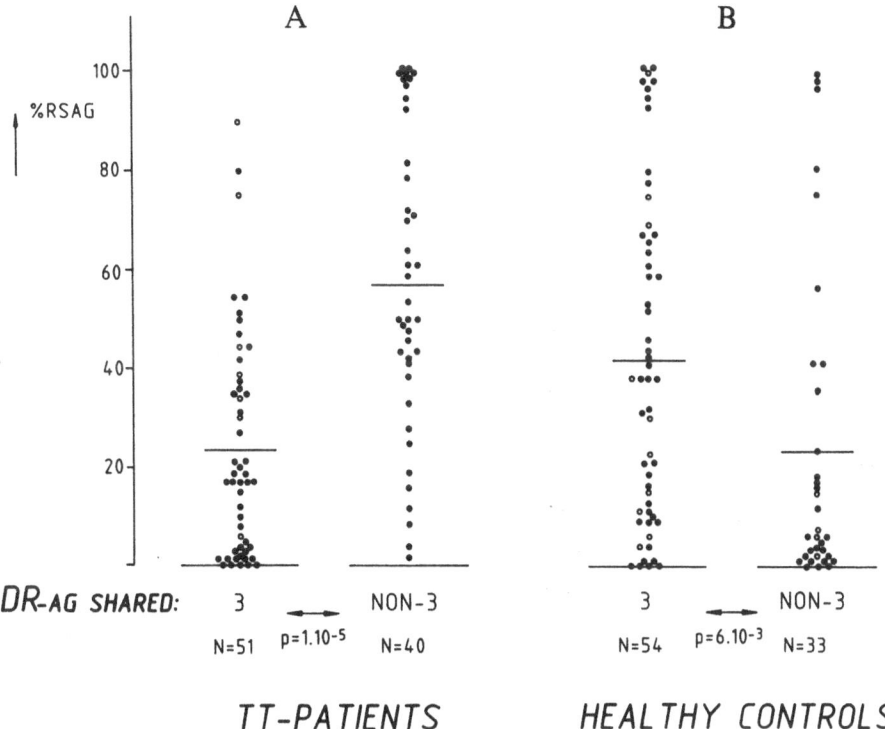

DR-AG SHARED:

TT-PATIENTS   HEALTHY CONTROLS

Fig. 4
A) Preferential HLA-DRnon3 restriction of *M. leprae* induced proliferation of TCL$_{lep}$ from 7 TT patients.
B) Preferential HLA-DR3 restriction of *M. leprae* induced proliferation of TCL$_{lep}$ from 8 healthy individuals.
See legend figure 3. Open circles in A) represent Surinam healthy control derived APC-patient TCL$_{lep}$ combinations; open circles in B) represent patient derived APC-Surinam healthy control TCL$_{lep}$ combinations.

preferentially DRnon3 restricted responsiveness of TCL$_{lep}$ in patients is *M. leprae* specific. PPD stimulated TCL$_{ppd}$ from three healthy controls showed the same preferential association of DR3 with responsiveness as the *M. leprae* stimulated TCL$_{lep}$ from these individuals (see above) as shown in the same figure (p=0.02). Mean responses in the DR3 shared group were 75.92±17.97% (n=12), and in the DRnon3 shared one 47.73±31.05% (n=11). Antigen specific T cell responses against PPD are known to be restricted by RDs associated with HLA-DR as previous studies have shown (e.g. ref. 11). Although we here have tested only 5 completely DR mismatched T cell-APC combinations for the 6 mentioned TCL$_{ppd}$, these results are consistent with a major role for DR as expected.
In summary, the induction of preferentially DRnon3 restricted T cell respon-

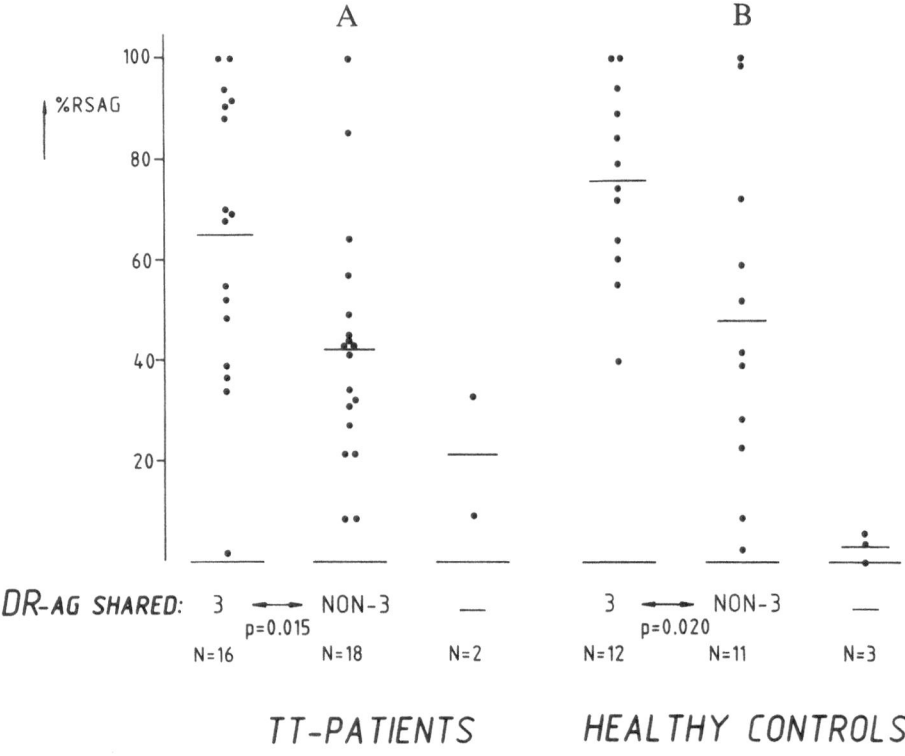

Fig. 5
Preferential HLA-DR3 restriction of PPD induced proliferation of TCL_{ppd} from 3 TT patients (A) and 3 healthy individuals (B). See legend figure 3. The 100% RSAG responses of these TLC were 12,100; 17,480; 20,155; 25,920; 26,540 and 78,560 cpm. Standard deviations did not exceed 15%.

sivensess against *M. leprae* in TT patients is *M. leprae* as well as patient specific since preferentially DR3 restricted responses against *M. tuberculosis* (PPD) are induced in TT patients, and since preferentially DR3 restricted responses against both *M. leprae* and *M. tuberculosis* are observed in healthy individuals.

M. leprae *specific induced preferential DRnon3 restriction of T cell responses of patients is crossreactive against other mycobacteria.*

Since the preferentially DRnon3 restricted responsiveness in TT patients was observed only for TCL_{lep} but not for TCL_{ppd} when tested against respectively *M. leprae* and PPD, we wanted to know whether or not the same phenomena would be observed when these TCL were tested against crossreactive antigens on other mycobacteria than those against the TCL has been raised, namely *M.*

113

leprae or PPD respectively. The results, depicted in figure 6, demonstrate that the *M. leprae* induced TCL_{lep} of 5 TT patients show the same preferentially DRnon3 restricted T cell responsiveness not only for *M. leprae*, but also for a series of other mycobacteria, including PPD. Conversely, *M. leprae* induced TCL_{lep} from 2 healthy controls as well as a PPD induced TCL_{ppd} from 1 TT patient show preferentially DR3 restricted responsiveness against virtually all mycobacteria tested. Note that TCL_{lep} from patients show a low response to PPD in association with DR3 in contrast to the TCL_{ppd} from these patients. Note in addition that the TCL_{ppd} from the only patient tested does not show DR3 associated lower responses to *M. leprae* in contrast to the TCL_{lep}.

In summary, the *M. leprae* or PPD induced preferentially DR3 or DRnon3 restricted T cell responsiveness is maintained when other crossreactive mycobacteria are presented to these T cells. Thus, as stated above the DRnon3 associated T cell responsiveness in patients is specifically induced by *M. leprae* but apparently is directed against crossreactive mycobacterial antigens.

M. leprae *reactive DR3 restricted T cell clones from TT patients may differ in antigen specificity and may be decreased in frequency in comparison to the DRnon3 restricted T cell clones.*

Because of the observed DR3 restricted *M. leprae* induced low T cell responsiveness in TT patients, we investigated whether quantitative or qualitative differences could be detected between *M. leprae* reactive T cell clones using either the DR3 or the DRnon3 molecules as restriction elements. T cell clones of such a TT patient were generated against *M. leprae*. The antigen specificity (8) and the HLA-DR encoded restriction determinants used by these helper T cell clones have been described recently (see chapter 5). A number of T cell clones recognized *M. leprae* in association with DR3 (n=8), whereas other clones used the other DR molecule (i.c. DR2) as restriction element (n=14). The frequency of DR3 restricted clones thus was lower (36%) than that of DRnon3 restricted ones (64%). Limiting dilution experiments also showed a twofold difference (data not shown).

Thus, although the same DR3 molecules which induce low TCL_{lep} responsiveness function as normal restriction elements for *M. leprae* reactive T cell clones of these same patients, such clones may be reduced in frequency. Apart from such quantitative differences in the frequencies of DR3 versus DRnon3 restricted clones, we also obtained evidence for qualitative differences between those two groups of clones. Whereas a similar frequency of DR3 as well as DRnon3 restricted clones was found to react with common mycobacterial antigens (DR3 restricted clones: n=4; DRnon3 restrictes ones: n=5), the DR3 restricted clones which are not reactive against common mycobacterial antigens recognize significantly more often *M. leprae* specific antigens than the DRnon3 restricted ones (see table II; p=0.02), suggesting a difference in antigen recognition repertoire. No differences were observed with regard to cell surface phenotypic markers or antigen induced γ-interferon production.

114

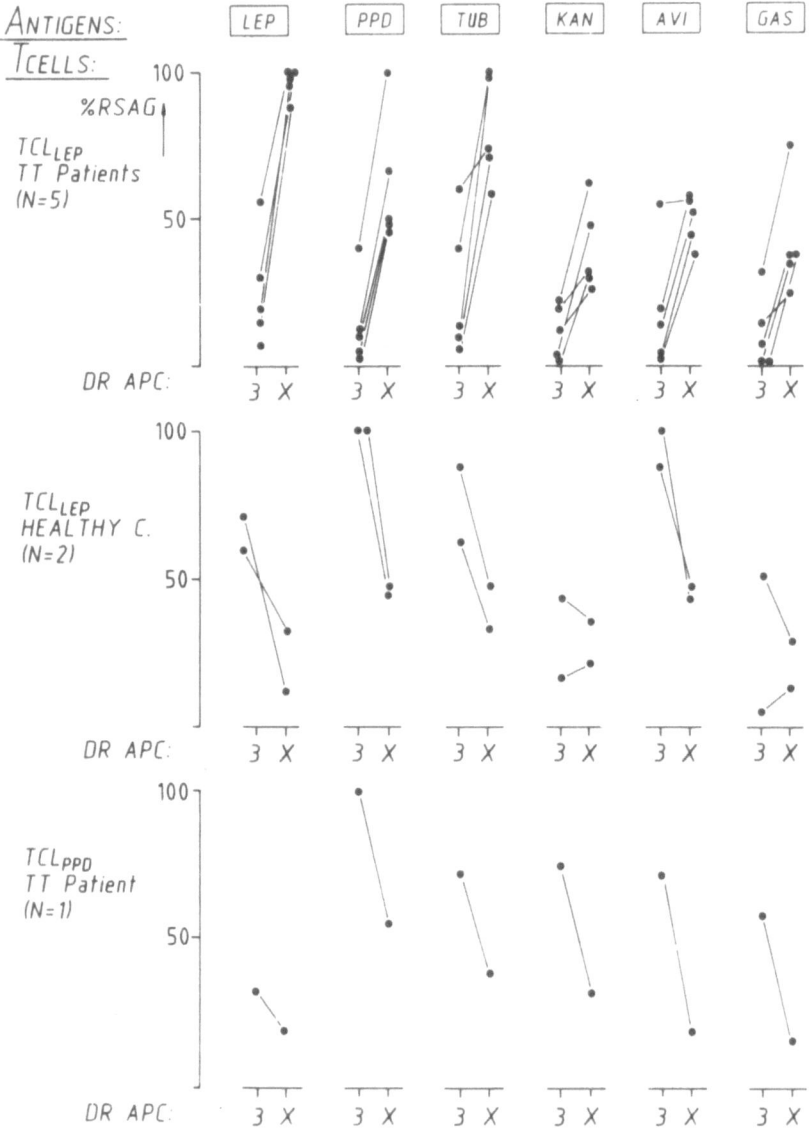

Fig. 6
The initially *M. leprae* or PPD induced preferential DRnon3 (DRx) or DR3 restriction of TCL from patients or controls is crossreactive against other mycobacterial antigens. The results for 5 TCL_{lep} from 5 TT patients, 2 TCL_{lep} from 2 healthy individuals and 1 TCL_{ppd} from a TT patient are expressed in %RSAG. Antigen was presented to each TCL via two allogeneic APC which shared respectively only the DR3 or the DRnon3 (x) with the T cell. To enable a comparison of the results for each individual TCL activated via DR3 or DRx, these two %RSAG's are connected for each antigen by a line. The antigens tested were: LEP: *M. leprae*; PPD; TUB: *M. tuberculosis*; KAN: *M. kansasii*; AVI: *M. avium*; GAS: *M. gastrii*. The 100% RSAG responses of the different TCL tested ranged between 10,955 and 50,713 cpm. Standard deviations were less than 15%.

115

Table II

Differences in *M. leprae* antigen recognition between DR3 and DRnon3 restricted T cell clones from a TT patient.

Antigen specificity* of T cell clones	*M. leprae* only	*M. leprae* and one – several myco-bacteria
Restriction determinant+ of T cell clones		
DR3	4	0
DRnon3°	2	7

$$p=0.02$$

* *M. leprae* antigens and other mycobacterial antigens were presented to cloned T cells from a TT patient as reported previously (18). The resulting antigen specificity patterns are shown.
+ The HLA-DR restriction specificities of the tested T cell clones were defined as described recently (chapter 5).
° The HLA class II phenotype of this patient was DR2, 3; DRw52; DQw1, 2; DPw5.

Preliminary evidence for preferentially DR3 restricted suppression of M. leprae *reactive helper T cells in TT patients.*

So far, we have defined the DR3 restricted *M. leprae* directed lower T cell responsiveness as being (i) confined to TT patients, (ii) induced specifically by *M. leprae*, (iii) crossreactive versus other mycobacteria, and (iv) not a consequence of the inability of DR3 molecules to present *M. leprae* to patients' T cells or the absence of DR3 restricted *M. leprae* reactive T cells in these patients, although such T cells may be decreased in frequency. However, apart from the latter observation, we still had no answer to the question why the DR3 restricted *M. leprae* induced T cell responsiveness was low. Therefore, we considered the possibility of suppressor T cells which might suppress such DR3 restricted *M. leprae* induced helper T cell responses.

We used the isolated DR3 or DRnon3 restricted *M. leprae* reactive helper T cell clones from one patient as probes for possible suppressor cells. *M. leprae* was presented to DR3 restricted clones (n=7) by DR3 homozygous APC and to DRnon3 restricted clones (n=7) by DRnon3 homozygous APC. To these respective cultures the (weakly irradiated (5 Gy)) autologous DR3/non3 TLC_{lep} was added. The addition of this TLC_{lep} led to suppression of the proliferative responses of most of the tested clones (figure 7). The mean suppression was 40.6%. Mean suppression of the DR2 restricted clones only was 26.6%, and of the DR3 restricted clones 54.7%. The DR3 restricted clones were suppressed more often (6 out of 7) above the average level of suppression when compared

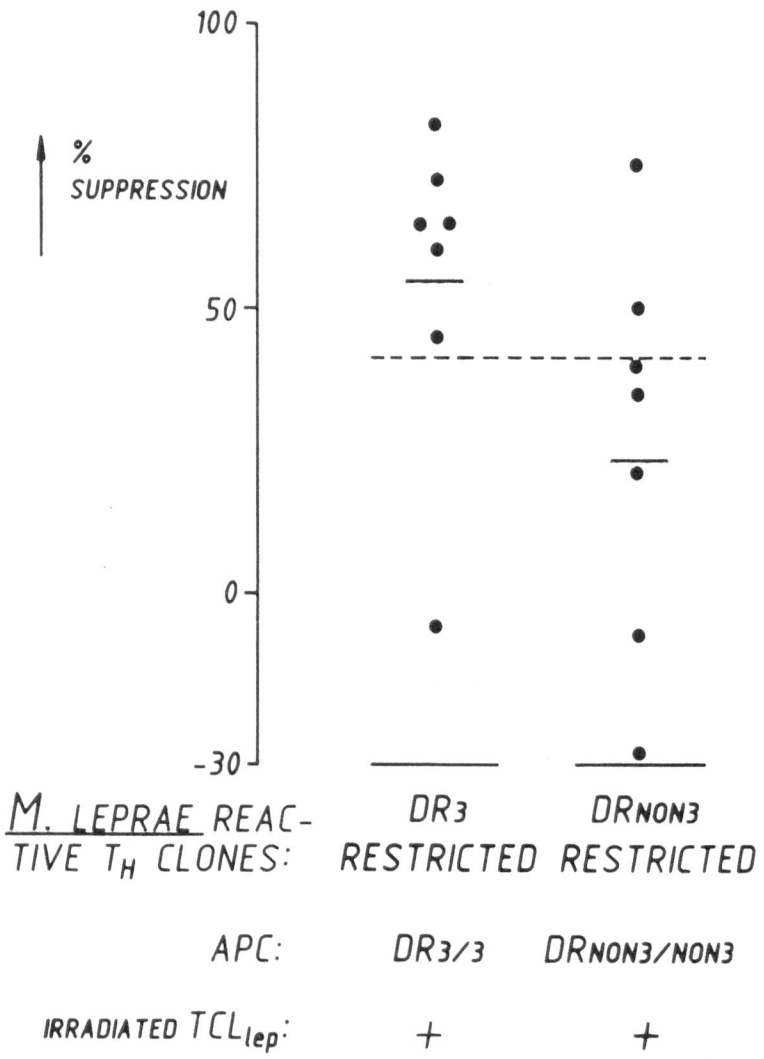

Fig. 7

M. leprae was presented to 7 DR3 restricted and to 7 DRnon3 restricted *M. leprae* reactive T cell clones (10^4 cells) from one TT patient respectively by either DR3 homozygous APC or by DRnon3 homozygous APC (5 x 10^4 cells; 40 Gy irradiated). Autologous TCL_{lep} cells were added to the cultures (10^5 cells) which did not proliferate anymore after irradiation (5 Gy). As a control, no TCL_{lep} cells were added. The results are expressed in % suppression, i.e. [1-(the observed proliferation in the presence of TCL_{lep} cells divided by the observed proliferation in the absence of TCL_{lep} cells] x 100% for each individual clone. The mean suppression for all clones was 40.6%, as indicated by the horizontal line, and for the DR3 or DR2 restricted clones 54.7% and 26.6% respectively as indicated. Proliferative responses of the DR3 restricted T cell clones were 11,315; 13,380; 18,560; 27,160; 30,165; 59,480 and 65,185 cpm; those of the DR2 restricted clones 4,513 , 4,890 , 13,175 , 16,210 , 20,075 , 34,425 and 50,650 cpm. Standard deviations did not exceed 10%.

to the DRnon3 restricted ones (2 out of 7). These results just reached the level of significance (p=0.05; Fisher's exact test).

Other experiments compatible with such a haplotype specificity of the observed suppression included mixing experiments in which both DR3 and DRnon3 APC were used to activate simultaneously a *M. leprae* reactive DR3/non 3 TCL_{lep} from a TT patient. The DRnon3 restricted responses were not influenced at all when presumably also the T cells restricted by the DR3 haplotype were activated. Thus, if these latter cells would include suppressor T cells, the suppression would be confined to the DR3 haplotype only.

These results may be interpreted as preliminar evidence for suppressor cells with a preference for DR3 restricted *M. leprae* helper T cells in patients. Sofar we have studied only one patient in this way. Clearly, it remains to be established whether this same tendency is observed in other patients as well and consequently whether these findings may be responsible in part of the DR3 associated lower *M. leprae* directed T cell responsiveness in patients.

Discussion

We have studied the association of HLA-DR3 with tuberculoid (TT) or high resistant leprosy in a Surinam population as a model for HLA class II regIr gene controlled susceptibility to disease. The results presented here indicate that DR3 molecules specifically differ from the DRnon3 ones with respect to their role in *M. leprae* specific T cell activation in TT leprosy patients. This DR3 specific difference suggests that the DR3 molecules are the products of a *M. leprae* specific HLA-DR3 regIr gene controlling the development of TT leprosy.

The previously (13) described association between DR3 and TT leprosy as compared to healthy controls and more significantly as compared to BL-LL patients was confirmed and extended. These data suggest that an HLA-DR3 associated regIr gene predisposes to TT leprosy which is characterized by relatively high T cell mediated immune reactivity against *M. leprae* but protects from BL-LL leprosy where T cell low- or non-responsiveness is observed. Similar evidence for such a role for DR3 has been collected in multicase leprosy family studies (20). The observation that in the 99 healthy individuals tested DR3 tends to protect from *in vitro* low- or nonresponsiveness against mycobacterial antigens, including *M. leprae* is consistent with the observed association with TT and not BL-LL leprosy as well as with the previously noted decreased frequency of DR3 among skin test nonresponders to mycobacteria including *M. leprae* (19; T.O. *et al.* submitted for publication).

The major evidence for a differential role of DR3 molecules in the immune response to *M. leprae* in relation with TT leprosy comes from the study of 345 allogeneic TCL_{lep}-APC combinations showing that HLA-DR molecules are the main restriction elements for T cell responses to *M. leprae* (this study; see chapter 5). Because TT leprosy correlates with *M. leprae* reactive T cell responsiveness, the DR3 associated regIr gene would be expected to control and regulate differentially T cell reactivity to *M. leprae*. Our data show that this is indeed the case: a *M. leprae* specific low T cell responsiveness was observed when TCL_{lep} from DR3/non3 heterozygous TT patients were activated by *M. leprae* plus allogeneic APC sharing only the DR3 with the TCL_{lep}; conversely, APC sharing only the DRnon3 with the TCL_{lep} induced high T cell responsiveness, thus confirming and extending significantly previous results of our group obtained with purified T cells and monocytes (21). The low T cell responsiveness observed in the present study is *M. leprae* specific, confined to TT patients and unique for DR3. This specific differential immune regulatory effect strongly suggests that DR3 molecules in these patients are the products of a *M. leprae* specific regIr gene which is associated with the development of TT leprosy.

It is interesting to note that in the case of both TCL_{lep} from healthy individuals as well as in the case of TCL_{ppd} from healthy individuals and TT patients a preferential DR3 restricted high responsiveness was found. This may be of relevance for the pathogenesis of TT leprosy, as will be discussed below.

To obtain more insight into the mechanism of the DR3 restricted *M. leprae* specific low T cell responsiveness in TT patients, we studied both APC and T cells as responsible cells for the regIr gene effect. No APC related DR3 associated defect in the presentation of *M. leprae* antigens could be detected, since the same DR3-APC which induced low TCL_{lep} responses in TT patients not only induced high TCL_{lep} responses in healthy individuals, but also could present *M. leprae* to patient derived *M. leprae* reactive T cell clones. There was also no general DR3 associated defect in antigen presentation to TCL of TT patients since DR3-APC could induce high TCL_{ppd} responses in these patients. Similarly, no significant differences were observed when patient and healthy control derived DR3-APC were compared with respect to their capacity to present *M. leprae* and other mycobacteria to TCL from patients and controls. Thus, an apparent defect expressed at the level of the APC which could be responsible for the observed DR3 restricted low responsiveness of TCL_{lep} in patients seems unlikely.

Studying then *M. leprae* induced T cell clones of a TT patient, it was observed that the frequency of DR3 restricted clones was approximately half of that of the DRnon3 restricted ones. Furthermore, the results indicated that DR3 restricted clones could be suppressed more often and more strongly by the autologous TCL_{lep} in the presence of DR3-APC than the DRnon3 restricted clones in the presence of DRnon3-APC suggesting the presence of DR3 haplotype related suppressor T cells. Although these findings quite clearly need to be extended to other TT patients before these observations may be generalized, at least they provide a rational explanation for the DR3 restricted low T cell responsiveness against *M. leprae* in TT leprosy. Another interesting observation may be that DR3 restricted clones apparently display another antigen recognition repertoire than the DRnon3 restricted ones. It is unknown whether -and if so, how- this difference in antigen specificity is related to the DR3-regIr gene and thus to TT leprosy.

The question which remains to be answered is how the *M. leprae* specific DR3 associated *low* responsiveness is related to TT leprosy, since one rather would expect *high* responsiveness to be associated with this form of leprosy. There are two possibilities: the observed low responsiveness either is directly related to the pathogenesis of TT leprosy or is a consequence of the development of TT leprosy. We consider the first possibility as an unlikely one since DR3 protects from and not predisposes to low- or non-responsiveness against mycobacteria *in vivo* (19, T.O. *et al.*, submitted for publication) and *in vitro* (vide supra). Moreover, whereas the DR3 restricted TCL_{lep} responsiveness in patients may be low, the DRnon3 restricted responses are high and thus would be dominant over the DR3 associated low responsiveness. This is also supported by the fact that such TT patients are good responders to *M. leprae* in skin testing and in lymphocyte transformation tests (7).

We postulate that the *M. leprae*-, TT- and DR3- specific low responsiveness is secondary to the development of TT leprosy, but that the DR3 associated regIr gene is etiologically related to TT leprosy. DR3 predisposes to (high) responsiveness against *M. leprae* and other mycobacteria. Only in genetically -non MHC controlled- or otherwise susceptible individuals, infection with *M. leprae* will be followed by the development of disease (8,9,20,22). When such susceptible individuals carry the DR3 associated regIr gene, (high) T cell responsiveness against *M. leprae* will develop which is preferentially restricted via the DR3 molecules. Whereas such (high) responsiveness on the one hand will protect against BL-LL leprosy, it may on the other hand easily lead to tissue damage and thus TT leprosy as a consequence of the apparently inappropriate regulation.

As soon as tissue damage occurs, the immune system then will develop a vigorous suppressive signal for these self destructive DR3 restricted T cells, as may be evidenced by the decreased frequency and the stronger suppression of such clones. The DR3 associated low responsiveness in TCL_{lep} of TT patients may well reflect this sequence of events. TT patients nevertheless do remain good responders to *M. leprae* via the DRnon3 molecules, since DRnon3 restricted T cells will not be suppressed by the DR3 specific suppressor cells. Thus, DR3 positive susceptible individuals will be and remain protected from developing BL-LL leprosy. Since healthy individuals are not susceptible to leprosy or tuberculosis and TT patients are resistant against the latter disease as well (7), the DR3 restricted high responsiveness in the respective TCL_{lep} and TCL_{ppd} from controls and the TCL_{ppd} from TT patients will not lead to tissue damage and consequently will remain high. It would be of interest to see whether DR3 restricted TCL_{lep} responses of TT patients before treatment or during the initial phase of the disease indeed are high, and become low later. So far, we have not been able to study such cases unfortunately.

The mechanism by which (high) *M. leprae* T cell responsiveness in susceptible individuals is related to the mentioned tissue damage in TT leprosy has not been understood fully. Peripheral nerve destruction is a common feature of TT leprosy. Nerve damage may be a nonspecific bystander effect of *M. leprae* triggered- inflammatory reactions in the proximity of such nerves, but may also represent true auto-immune responsiveness to nerve tissue antigens. This latter possibility is supported by experimental studies in which TT leprosy-like lesions could be induced in rabbits and rats upon immunization with peripheral nerve antigen (23,24). Such antigens may be exposed after *M. leprae*-mediated damage of Schwann cells or other nerve components. Another possibility is antigenic mimicry between *M. leprae* and nerve antigens: the DR3 restricted *M. leprae* reactive T cells from susceptible (TT) individuals would then preferentially recognize antigens on *M. leprae* that are also expressed by self nerve-tissue. A temporary break of self-tolerance would then lead to auto-immune reactions against self-nerve antigens. In experimental animals, auto-immunity may be triggered by antigenic mimicry between self and microbial components (e.g. 25,26). Along this line, monoclonal antibodies specific for mycobacteria have been found to crossreact with human tissue antigens (27). It may be relevant that the DR3 restricted clones recognize other *M. leprae* antigens then the DRnon3 restricted ones. Future studies should address whether these DR3 restricted clones crossreact with e.g. nerve antigens.

The postulated predisposition to tissue damage and thus TT leprosy as a consequence of inappropriate DR3 controlled T cell responsiveness against *M. leprae* antigens is consistent with a number of experimental animal studies. Such a role for vigorously responding antigen specific helper T cells in susceptibility to disease triggered by micro-organisms has been shown in mice, genetically susceptible for *Leishmania major*, a protozoan parasite. The transfer of *L. major* specific helper T cells strongly enhanced the development of cutaneous lesions induced by the parasite (28). *In vivo* treatment with an anti L3T4 ("helper" T cell subset) monoclonal antibody resulted in a drastic resolution of the lesions (29). In other studies, antibodies against H-2I (the murine MHC class II) antigens modified the formation of granulomata during *Schistosoma mansoni* infection (30). H-2 linked genes indeed control the development of granulomatous lesions upon infection, as has been shown for *M. lepraemurium* (31,32).

A lack of control in DR3 associated immune reactivity has been observed in a variety of systems (e.g. 33-37), including reactivity against auto-antigens such as the acetylcholine receptor in myasthenia gravis patients (33), and may be consistent with the mentioned associations between DR3 and auto-immune like diseases.

Finally, it is interesting that a similar DR3 associated low T cell responsiveness has been described for the gluten antigen, the triggering antigen of celiac disease. This disease is associated with DR3 and DR7 (38). The frequency of both DR3 and DR7 restricted gluten specific T cells was decreased as compared to the DRnon3-non7 restricted ones (39). Similar findings were reported by the same investigators for mumps and Coxsackie-B4 virus in healthy controls and in type I diabetes mellitus patients, where also the DR3 antigen is increased in frequency (40). The fact however that these findings were not confined to patients only

121

but observed in healthy individuals as well suggests that other immunoregulatory DR3 associated mechanisms may be operative there, and thus that multiple DR3 associated regIr gene mechanisms exist.

Summary

The type of leprosy that develops upon infection correlates with the helper T (Th) cell mediated immune reactivity against *Mycobacterium leprae* which is high in tuberculoid (TT) but low or absent in lepromatous (BL-LL) leprosy. The TT but not the BL-LL type of leprosy is associated with HLA-DR3 in a Surinam population. Thus, a DR3 associated immune regulation (regIr) gene may predispose to TT leprosy by regulating Th cell activity against *M. leprae*. We here report a differential role for DR3 versus other DR (non3) products in Th cell responsiveness against *M. leprae* and related antigens, both in TT patients and in healthy individuals. The results show that: (i) DR3 tended to protect against nonresponsiveness against mycobacterial antigens in healthy individuals (n=99) as measured by lymphocyte transformation tests (p=0.05); (ii) Th cell responses of *M. leprae* induced Th cell lines (TCL$_{lep}$) of healthy controls as well as TT patients were mainly HLA-DR restricted (studied in resp. 148 (p=3x10^{-4}) and 197 (p=10^{-6}) allogeneic Th cell-APC (antigen presenting cell) combinations); DR3 was associated with *high* Th cell responsiveness when in DR3/non3 heterozygous healthy controls (n=8) the DR3 restricted responses of TCL$_{lep}$ were compared with the DRnon3 restricted ones in respectively 54 and 33 allogeneic Th cell-APC (p=6x10^{-3}); in contrast DR3 was associated with *low* Th cell responsiveness in DR3/non3 heterozygous TT patients (n=7) when similar (resp. 51 and 40) Th cell-APC combinations were studied (p= 10^{-5}); (iii) DR3 was associated with *high* Th cell responsiveness against *M. tuberculosis* (PPD) in the same TT patients (n=3) as well as in healthy controls (n=3), studied in resp. 26 and 36 combinations (resp. p=0.015 and p=0.020); (iv) the DR3 associated *low* TCL$_{lep}$ responsiveness in TT patients is induced by *M. leprae* specific antigens, but -once induced- is directed against common mycobacterial antigens; the DR3 associated high responsiveness of TCL$_{ppd}$ from patients and of TCL$_{lep}$ from healthy individuals similarly is directed against common antigens on mycobacteria; (v) DR3 restricted *M. leprae* reactive cloned T cells from a TT patient were found to recognize other antigenic determinants on the bacillus and were suppressed more often and more strongly by autologous T cells than the DRnon3 restricted clones; such a haplotype related suppression may account for the DR3 associated *low* responsiveness of TCL$_{lep}$ in TT leprosy.

The study presented here has enabled us to identify DR3 as the product of a *M. leprae* specific DR3 associated regIr gene, and to study the role of DR3 in the regulation of the immune response against *M. leprae*. Thus, this study may provide a model for the unravelling of the mechanism of other HLA class II-disease associations.

122

Acknowledgements

We wish to thank Dr. P. Niemel (Rotterdam), and the staff members at the Dermatology Departments of the University Hospital of Amsterdam, the Dijkzigt Hospital in Rotterdam and the University Hospital of Paramaribo for their generous help in collecting blood samples. Furthermore we thank Dr. R.C. Good, Atlanta, for supplying us with Dharmendra's antigen, Paul Klatser for mycobacterial antigens, Joe D'Amaro and Peter de Lange for statistical advice and Tiny van Westerop for preparing the manuscript. This study was supported in part by the Foundation for Medical Research (MEDIGON; grant nr. 900-509-099), the Immunology of Leprosy (IMMLEP) component of the UNDP/WORLD Bank/WHO Special Programme for Research and Training in Tropical Diseases, the Netherlands Leprosy Relief Association (NSL) and the J.A. Cohen Institute for Radiopathology and Radiation Protection (IRS).

References

1. Benacerraf, B. 1981. Role of MHC gene products in immune regulation. Science 212: 1229.
2. Schwartz, R.H. 1986. Immune response (Ir) genes of the murine major histocompatibility complex. Adv. Immunol. 38: 31.
3. Janeway, C.A. 1983. Immune response genes, the problem of the non responder, a commentary on. The Ia molecule of the antigen presenting cell plays a critical role in immune response gene regulation of T cell activation. J. Mol. Cell. Immunol. 1: 15.
4. Sasazuki, T., Nishimura, Y., Muto, M. and Ohta, N. 1983. HLA-linked genes controlling immune response and disease susceptibility. Immunol. Rev. 70: 51.
5. Hensen, E. and Elferink, B.G. 1984. The immune response to (T,G)-A-L and GAT in man: an association of non-responsiveness to (T,G)-A-L with HLA-DRw8. Hum. Immunol. 10:113.
6. Ottenhoff, T.H.M., Torres, P, Terencio de las Aguas, J., Fernandez, R., van Eden, W., de Vries, R.R.P. and Stanford, J.L. 1986. Evidence for an HLA-DR4 associated immune response gene for *Mycobacterium tuberculosis*: a clue to the pathogenesis of rheumatoid arthritis? Lancet ii: 310
7. Bloom, B.R. and Godal, T. 1983. Selective primary health care: strategies for control of disease in the developing world. V. Leprosy. Rev. Infect. Dis. 5: 765.
8. Van Eden, W. and de Vries, R.R.P. 1984. HLA and leprosy: a re-evaluation. Lepr. Rev. 55: 89.
9. Serjeantson, S.W. 1983. HLA and susceptibility to leprosy. Immunol. Rev. 70: 89
10. De Vries, R.R.P., van Eden, W. and Ottenhoff, T.H.M. 1985. HLA class II immune response genes and products in leprosy. Progr. Allergy 36: 95.
11. Ottenhoff, T.H.M., Elferink, B.G., Hermans, J. and de Vries, R.R.P. 1985. HLA class II restriction repertoire of antigen specific T cells. I. The main restriction determinants for antigen presentation are associated with HLA-D/DR and not with DP and DQ. Hum. Immunol. 13: 105.
12. Ridley, D.S. and Jopling, W.H. 1966. Classification of leprosy according to immunity. A five-group system. Int. J. Lepr. 34: 255.
13. Van Eden, W., de Vries, R.R.P., D'Amaro, J., Schreuder, G.M.Th., Leiker, D.L. and van Rood,J.J. 1982. HLA-DR associated genetic control of the type of leprosy in a population from Surinam. Hum. Immunol. 4: 343.
14. Van Leeuwen, A. and van Rood, J.J. 1980. Description of B-cell methods. In:*Histocompatibility Testing 1980* (ed. Terasaki, P.I.), Los Angeles, UCLA Press, p. 278.
15. Van Rood, J.J. 1979. Microlymphocytotoxicity method. In:*Manual of Tissue Typing Techniques*(ed. Ray, J.G.), National Institutes of Health, Bethesda, MD. p. 104.
16. Svejgaard, A., Jersild, C., Staub Nielsen, L. and Bodmer,W.F. 1974. HLA antigens and disease. Statistical and general considerations. Tissue Antigens 4: 94.
17. Haanen, J.B.A.G., Ottenhoff,T.H.M., Voordouw, A., Elferink, B.G., Klatser, P.R., Spits, H.and de Vries, R.R.P. 1986. HLA class II restricted *Mycobacterium leprae* reactive T cell clones from leprosy patients established with a minimal requirement for autologous mononuclear cells. Scand. J. Immunol. 23: 101.
18. Ottenhoff, T.H.M., Klatser, P.R., Ivanyi, J., Elferink, B.G., de Wit, M.Y.L. and de Vries, R.R.P. 1986. *Mycobacterium leprae* specific protein antigens defined by cloned human helper T cells. Nature 319: 66.
19. Van Eden, W., de Vries, R.R.P., Stanford, J.L. and Rook, G.A.W. 1982. HLA-DR3 associated genetic control of response to multiple skin tests with new tuberculins. Clin. Exp. Immunol.52: 287.
20. Van Eden, W., Gonzalez, N.M., de Vries, R.R.P., Convit, J. and van Rood, J.J. 1985. HLA-linked control of predisposition to lepromatous leprosy. J. Infect. Dis. 151: 9.
21. Van Eden, W., Elferink, B.G., de Vries, R.R.P., Leiker, D.L. and van Rood, J.J. 1984. Low T-lymphocyte responsiveness to *Mycobacterium leprae* antigens in association with HLA-DR3. Clin. Exp. Immunol. 55: 140.

124

22. Xu Keju, de Vries, R.R.P., Fei Hongming, van Leeuwen, A., Chen Renbiao and Ye Ganyun. 1985. HLA-linked control of predisposition to lepromatous leprosy. Int. J. Lepr. 53: 56.
23. Crawford, C.L., Evans, D.H.L. and Evans, E.M. 1974. Experimental allergic neuritis induced by sensory nerve myelin may provide a model for non-lepromatous leprosy. Nature 251: 223.
24. Crawford, C.L., Hardwicke, P.M.D., Evans, D.H.L. and Evans, E.M. 1977. Granulomatous hypersensitivity induced by sensory peripheral nerve. Nature 265: 457.
25. Van Eden, W., Holoshitz, J. Nevo, Z., Frenkel, A., Klajman, A. and Cohen, I.R. 1985. Arthritis induced by a T-lymphocyte clone that responds to *Mycobacterium tuberculosis* and to cartilage proteoglycans. Proc. Natl. Acad. Sci. USA 82: 5117.
26. Jahnke, U., Fisher, E.H. and Alrond, E.C. 1985. Sequence homology between certain viral proteins and proteins related to encephalomyelitis and neuritis. Science 229: 282.
27. Thorns, C.J. and Morris, J.A. 1985. Common epitopes between mycobacterial and certain host tissue antigens. Clin. Exp. Immunol. 61: 323.
28. Titus, R.G., Lima, G.C., Engers, H.D. and Louis, J.A. 1984. Exacerbation of murine cutaneous leishmaniasis by adoptive transfer of parasite-specific helper T cell populations capable of mediating *Leishmania major* - specific delayed type hypersensitivity. J. Immunol. 133: 1594.
29. Titus, R.G., Ceredig, R., Cerottini, J. and Louis, J.A. 1985. Therapeutic effect of anti-L3T4 monoclonal antibody GK 1.5 on cutaneous leishmaniasis in genetically susceptible BALB/c mice. J. Immunol. 135: 2108.
30. Green, W.F. and Colley, D.G. 1981. Modulation of *Schistosoma mansoni* egg-induced granuloma formation: I-J restriction of T-cell mediated suppression in a chronic parasitic infection. Proc.Natl. Acad. Sci. USA 78: 1152.
31. Closs, O. Løvik, M., Wigzell, H. and Taylor, B.A. 1983. H-2 linked gene(s) influence the granulomatous reaction to viable *Mycobacterium lepraemurium* in the mouse. Scand. J. Immunol.18: 59.
32. Adu, H.O., Curtis, J. and Turk, J.L. 1983. Role of the major histocompatibility complex in resistance and granuloma formation in response to *Mycobacterium lepraemurium* infection. Infect.Immun. 40: 720.
33. Hohlfeld, R., Toyka, K.V., Heininger, K., Grosse-Wilde, H. and Kalies, I. 1984. Auto-immune human T lymphocytes specific for acetyl choline receptor. Nature 310: 244.
34. Pozzilli, P., Tarn, A.C. and Gale, E.A.M. 1985. HLA-DR3 and activated lymphocytes: significance in auto-immunity. Lancet ii: 954.
35. Ambinder, J.M., Chiorazzi, N. Gibofsky, A., Fotino, M. and Kunkel, H.G. 1982. Special characteristics of cellular immune function in normal individuals of the HLA-DR3 type. Clin.Immunol. Immunopathol. 23: 269.
36. Pollack, M.S., Vugrin, D., Hennessy, W., Herr, H.W., Dupont, B. and Whitmore, W.F. 1982. HLA antigens in patients with germ cell cancer of the testis. Cancer Res. 42: 2470.
37. Singal, D.P. and Fagnilli, L. 1982. Proliferation of alloantigen sensitized human peripheral blood lymphocytes by autologous cells associated with the HLA-B8/DR3. Clin. Exp. Immunol.49: 652.
38. Svejgaard, A., Platz, P. and Ryder, L.P. 1983. HLA and disease 1982 - a survey. Immunol.Rev. 70: 193.
39. Scott, H., Hirschberg, H. and Thorsby, E. 1983. HLA-DR3 and HLA-DR7 - restricted T cell hyporesponsiveness to gluten antigen: a clue to the aetiology of coeliac disease? Scand. J. Immunol.18: 163.
40. Bruserud, Ø., Stenersen, M. and Thorsby, E. 1985. T. lymphocyte response to Coxsackie B4 and mumps virus. II. Immunoregulation by HLA-DR3 and -DR4 associated restriction elements. Tissue Antigens 26: 179.

CHAPTER 8

EVIDENCE FOR AN HLA-DR4 ASSOCIATED IMMUNE RESPONSE GENE FOR *MYCOBACTERIUM TUBERCULOSIS*: A CLUE TO THE PATHOGENESIS OF RHEUMATOID ARTHRITIS?*

Summary

Skin test responses against mycobacterial antigens were studied in 86 Caucasoid leprosy patients after the intradermal injection of respectively *Mycobacterium tuberculosis*, *M. leprae*, *M. scrofulaceum* and *M. vaccae* antigens. The height of the responses (in mm of induration at 72 hours) was analyzed in relationship with the HLA class II phenotypes of the individuals tested. HLA-DR4 was associated with high responsiveness against the *M. tuberculosis* specific but not the common antigens shared with other mycobacteria (p = 0.0005). Because DR4 is associated with rheumatoid arthritis (RA) and because a role for *M. tuberculosis* antigens has been suggested both in experimentally induced auto-immune arthritis in rats and in RA, the observed DR4 associated regulation of the *in vivo* immune response against *M. tuberculosis* may well be relevant for the pathogenesis of RA.

Introduction

The class II region of the major histocompatibility complex (MHC) contains immune response (Ir) genes, the products of which are the MHC class II molecules (1). These MHC class II Ir genes are known to control immune responsiveness against T cell dependent foreign antigens (2). The extensive polymorphism of the class II Ir genes and molecules results in genetically controlled interindividual differences in antigen specific immune responsiveness. This in turn may lead to differential susceptibility to or expression of disease (2-4). The observed associations between HLA (the human MHC) class II antigens and several – mostly auto-immune – diseases are assumed to reflect such Ir gene controlled differences in antigen specific immune responsiveness (4). However, the supposed exogenous or endogenous triggering antigens for these diseases have remained unknown, with the exception of leprosy and celiac disease (5-7).

* Tom H.M. Ottenhoff, Pedro Torres, José Terencio de las Aguas, Ramon Fernandez, Willem van Eden, René R.P. de Vries and John L. Stanford. 1986. Lancet ii: 310-313.

Previous work has shown that HLA class II antigens are associated with genetically controlled differences in delayed type hypersensitivity (DTH) skin test responses to *Mycobacterium leprae* in leprosy patients (8; T.O. *et al*, submitted for publication). Moreover, HLA-DR3 was found to protect against responsiveness to mycobacterial antigens in healthy British individuals (9). In the present study, skin test responses against four related mycobacteria were investigated in leprosy patients, mainly of the lepromatous type, from Spain. The fact that the majority of these patients displays a specific nonresponsiveness to antigens expressed by *M. leprae* (10) offers a good possibility to study skin test responses against specific antigens expressed by other mycobacteria but not *M. leprae*.

We now report that HLA-DR4 is associated with high skin test responsiveness against *M. tuberculosis* specific antigens. The possible relevance of this finding for the pathogenesis of rheumatoid arthritis (RA) is discussed.

Patients and methods

Patients

Eighty-six unrelated Spanish leprosy patients were selected at random from the Sanatorio San Francisco de Borja, Fontilles in Alicante, Spain. Eight of them had been classified as (borderline) tuberculoid leprosy patients whereas 77 patients had been classified as (borderline) lepromatous leprosy cases, according to the five-group system described by Ridley and Jopling (11). The diagnosis was based on regular and careful clinical examination, review of the clinical histories, skin-slit smear bacteriology, histo-pathological examination of skin biopsy specimens and lepromin skin test reactivity. One patient could only be classified as an indeterminate leprosy case. All patients had received regular anti-leprosy multi drug treatment for several years.

Skin testing

Soluble preparations of ultrasonicates ("new tuberculins") of respectively *Mycobacterium tuberculosis*, *M. leprae*, *M. scrofulaceum* and *M. vaccae* which had been standardized according to their protein concentration (2 $\mu g/ml$) by spectrophotometry were used as skin test reagents in the way described previously (12, 13). In brief, 0.1 ml of each preparation was injected separately into the dermis of the volar surface of the forearm at the same time, 2 on each arm. Responses were recorded as mean diameters (in mm) of induration 72 hours after injection.

HLA-typing

Typing for the HLA-DR specificities was performed with 80 platelet absorbed sera in the two colour fluorescence test as described previously (14,15).

Statistical analysis

The significance of the differences in the distribution of the skin-test results for the different HLA-DR antigens were determined by the nonparametric Mann-Whitney rank sum test (SPSS-X computer package). This was done by calculating the significance of the difference in the distribution of the skin test results for each antigenic preparation between respectively those individuals with a particular DR specificity (DRx) and those without that specificity (DRnonx).

Results

The results of the skin tests obtained with each of the four different mycobacterial antigens were analyzed against the HLA-DR phenotypes of the 86 individuals tested. The results of these comparisons are shown in table I. HLA-

Table I.

Statistical significance of the influence of individual HLA-DR specificities on mycobacterial antigen induced skin test responses

HLA class II		(N_1=..;N_2=...)	Mycobacteria tested:			
specificities analyzed			*M.tuberculosis*	*M.leprae*	*M. scrofulaceum*	*M. vaccae*
N_1	N_2					
DR 1 ⟷ non 1		(15;71)	0.17	0.90	0.82	0.94
2 ⟷ non 2		(30;55)	0.78	0.72	0.54	1.00
3 ⟷ non 3		(13;72)	0.29	0.66	0.69	0.38
4 ⟷ non 4		(11;74)	0.0005	0.29	0.90	0.31
5 ⟷ non 5		(27;57)	0.74	0.66	0.80	0.56
w6 ⟷ non 6		(20;65)	0.73	0.73	0.82	0.93
7 ⟷ non 7		(27;58)	0.76	0.64	0.73	0.24
w8 ⟷ non 8		(5;81)	0.23	0.09	0.06	0.21
w9 ⟷ non 9		(1;85)	0.17	0.74	0.09	0.11
w10 ⟷ non 10		(4;82)	0.13	0.52	0.31	0.35

The differences in the distribution of the skin test results for the four mycobacterial antigens tested between those individuals (n=86) with a particular DR specificity (DRx; see column N_1) and those without that specificity (DRnonx; see column N_2) were analyzed by the Mann Whitney rank sum test. The resulting p-values are given. N_1 refers to the number of DRx positive individuals whereas N_2 refers to the number of the corresponding DRnonx individuals. Whenever N_1+N_2< 86 for a certain DR specificity, this was due to the fact that in the missing cases the presence or absence of that specificity could not be determined with certainty. Those cases were excluded from the analysis for that DR-specificity.

DR4 appeared to be associated with high responsiveness against *M. tuberculosis* (p= 0.0005), but not against the other three mycobacterial species. This finding remains significant when corrected for the number of comparisons made, i.e. 40 (10 DR specificities times 4 mycobacterial antigens) (p$_c$ = 0.02). The actual data obtained from the *M. tuberculosis* skin tests in respectively the DR4 and DRnon4 individuals are shown in figure 1. The association of DR4 with high responsiveness against *M. tuberculosis* was not caused by the presence of 23 *M. tuberculosis* nonresponders (0 mm) in the DRnon4 individuals (see figure 1) since an analysis restricted to the *M. tuberculosis* responders ($\geq$ 5 mm) revealed a similar difference (p= 0.005; n$_{DR4}$= 11, n$_{DRnon4}$= 51).

The association between DR4 and high skin test responsiveness to *M. tuberculosis* indeed seemed to be specific for *M. tuberculosis*, as further analysis of the skin test responses to *M. scrofulaceum* and *M. vaccae* confirmed: 10 patients responded to *M. scrofulaceum* and not to *M. vaccae*, 7 to *M. vaccae* and not to *M. scrofulaceum* and 16 to both of these antigens. In the *M. scrofulaceum* responders (n=26), 4 patients were DR4 positive whereas in the *M. vaccae* responders (n=23) 5 patients carried the DR4 specificity. In neither of these 2 responder groups (thus neglecting the nonresponders as was also done for *M. tuberculosis*) an association of DR4 with high responsiveness was observed, in contrast to the above mentioned results for the *M. tuberculosis* responder group.

As shown in figure 1, the association of DR4 with high *M. tuberculosis* responsiveness was also not caused by a non-random distribution of tuberculoid (marked by open circles) versus lepromatous patients (closed circles), since this association was observed in both groups of patients (respectively p = 0.05 and p = 0.003).

Of the 5 DRw8 positive patients, 2 had tuberculoid and one indeterminate leprosy. The overrepresentation of non-lepromatous patients in this group explains the tendency towards higher *M. leprae* skin test responsiveness as compared to the DRnon8.

As expected, skin test responses against *M. leprae* were absent in the majority of the lepromatous patients (66 of the 77; including 7 of the 8 DR4 positive patients) in contrast to the 8 tuberculoid patients, only one of which showed no response to *M. leprae*.

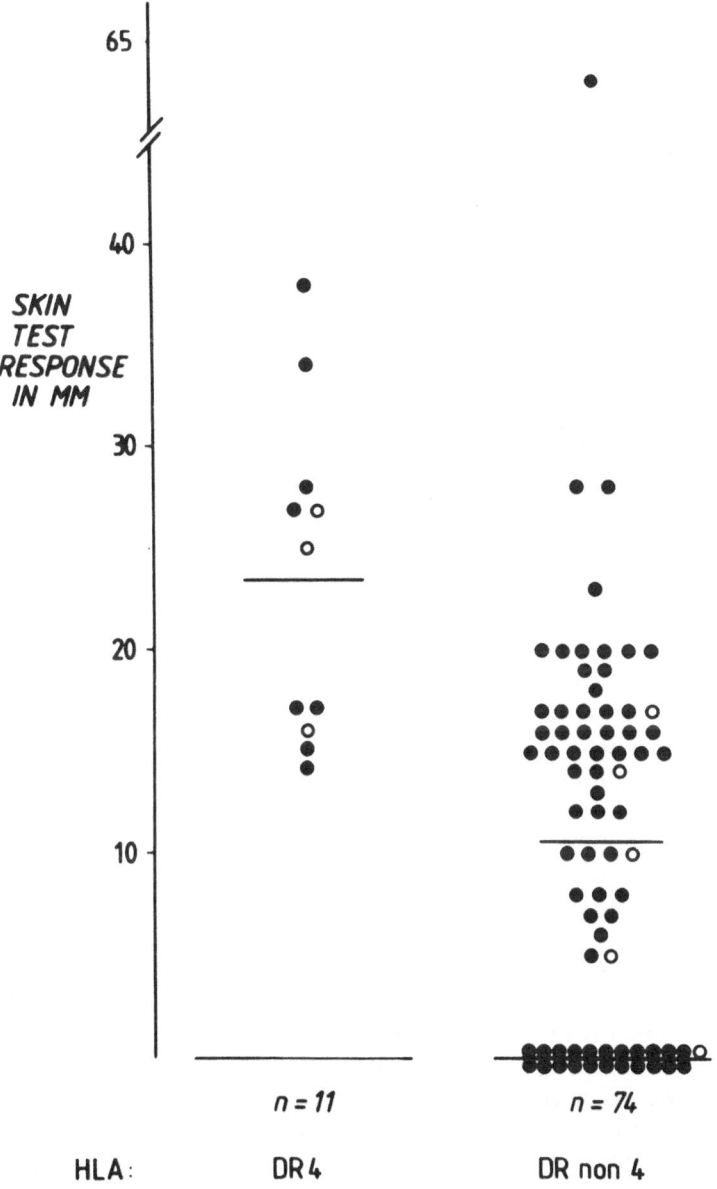

Fig. 1
HLA-DR4 associated high skin test responsiveness against *Mycobacterium tuberculosis* antigens in Spanish leprosy patients. Tuberculoid patients are indicated with open circles, lepromatous ones with closed ones. Mean responses for DR4 positive individuals were 23.45 mm, and for DRnon4 individuals 10.57 mm and are marked in the figure.

Discussion

In the 86 individuals studied here, HLA-DR4 is associated with high skin test responsiveness against *M. tuberculosis* (p = 0.0005) but not against *M. leprae*, *M. scrofulaceum* and *M. vaccae*. Since all four mycobacteria carry the common mycobacterial antigens (16) and since in addition *M. tuberculosis* and *M. scrofulaceum* share the "slow grower" antigens (16), we conclude that DR4 is associated with high responsiveness against (a) species specific antigen(s) of *M. tuberculosis*.

This conclusion may also be supported by the fact that the majority (77%) of the individuals tested here were lepromatous leprosy patients, showing the characteristic (skin test) nonresponsiveness against *M. leprae* (10). This unresponsiveness must include both the specific and the common antigens present on the leprosy bacillus (17). Such patients probably then remain responders against the species specific determinants of other mycobacteria, since this latter group of antigens is not shared with *M. leprae*, and therefore will not be involved in this nonresponsiveness. An alternative explanation for the *M. leprae* specific unresponsiveness would be the presence of a dominant *M. leprae* specific immunosuppression inducing epitope affecting (skin test) responses against both the species specific and the common antigens of *M. leprae*. In that case, responses against the common antigens on other mycobacteria would remain unaffected in the absence of such a *M. leprae* specific suppression inducing determinant. However, dominant suppression inducing epitopes affecting skin test responses have thusfar only been recognized in certain fast growing mycobacterial species (18), but not in the case of *Mycobacterium leprae* (19).

Thus, in the population studied here HLA-DR4 is a marker for an HLA class II Ir gene for *M. tuberculosis* specific antigens, conferring skin test high responsiveness. Since such DTH-type skin test responses are predominantly mediated by antigen specific helper T lymphocytes (20), and since such T lymphocytes recognize antigen only in association with a class II molecule, a phenomenon known as class II restriction (21), class II Ir gene products probably control such T cell mediated immune responses by regulating antigen specific helper T cell activation. In experimental animal models, such an Ir gene controlled T cell activation has been clearly demonstrated in different systems (e.g. 2, 23-25). In the only two HLA class II-associated diseases in which the triggering foreign antigen is known, similar evidence has been presented, namely for leprosy (3) and celiac disease (6).

Thus, in these animal and human disease models, class II Ir gene controlled antigen specific T cell activation explains the *in vivo* observed association of that class II Ir gene product with the disease. The known HLA class II antigens are markers for these Ir gene products.

Rheumatoid arthritis (RA) is a disease which is remarkably associated with HLA-DR4 (e.g. 26). Evidence from experimental animal models has suggested a role for *M. tuberculosis* antigens in the pathogenesis of RA: auto-immune arthritis

(AA) can be induced in MHC susceptible rats by inoculation with *M. tuberculosis* (23) and AA can be transferred to naive animals by *M. tuberculosis* specific T lymphocyte clones (28) from inoculated rats. Such arthritogenic T lymphocyte clones have been shown to crossreact between *M. tuberculosis* and proteoglycan components of joint cartilage, suggesting structural mimicry between *M. tuberculosis* and these auto-antigens (29). Of interest in this respect are recent observations made with cloned T cells which had been derived from the synovial fluid from affected joints of RA patients: such T cells also showed reactivity against *M. tuberculosis* antigens (30, 31). This suggests that the AA model may be extrapolated to RA: *M. tuberculosis* antigens may be relevant in the pathogenesis of RA, and this may be reflected in the association of DR4 with both RA and high responsiveness against *M. tuberculosis* specific antigens. This could be compatible with an earlier hypothesis, suggesting that RA is a disease with disturbed T cell-macrophage immunoregulation (32).

Although it is quite obvious that more evidence is necessary before the link between DR4, RA and high responsiveness against *M. tuberculosis* has been established, our findings at least provide a new clue for the rational search for such an antigen specific disease related class II Ir gene. Such findings may be important for the understanding of the mechanism of HLA-disease associations. It is clear that similar skin test studies have now to be performed in other populations, including healthy controls and RA patients. In previous skin test studies (e.g. 33, 34) in RA patients as well as in healthy controls, only one mycobacterial antigen was tested (PPD), so that no conclusions could be drawn as to the possible mycobacterial antigen specificity of these responses. Although in these studies skin test responses in RA patients were found to be non-specifically suppressed relative to those in healthy controls, antigen specific differences nevertheless might still be distinguishable. It therefore remains an intriguing question whether DR4 is also associated with high *M. tuberculosis* specific skin test responses in these two groups of individuals. Since both healthy controls and RA patients will probably - in addition to the species specific antigens - also respond to the common antigens, the DR4-Ir gene effect for *M. tuberculosis* specific antigens observed in leprosy patients may well be masked. In that case, a preparation containing only the *M. tuberculosis* species specific and not the common antigenic determinants should be tested. Apart from such responses to other than the species specific antigens of *M. tuberculosis* in addition also secondary immunoregulation in RA patients as a possible consequence of the development of RA might obscure the postulated initial high responsiveness that led to the development of tissue damage and thus disease. In the mentioned rat model, inoculation with *M. tuberculosis* not only induced T cells that caused AA, but also another subpopulation of T cells that could prevent or reverse the development of AA, albeit only upon transfer to other animals. These protective T cells have been found to induce anti-idiotypic suppression that is non-specific in its effector phase, thus suppressing non-related T cells as well (I.R. Cohen, personal communication). Such a mechanism could (partially)

132

account for the repeatedly observed general impairment of cell mediated immune responsiveness in RA patients as compared to healthy controls (33, 34). Another model for secondary immunoregulation may be tuberculoid leprosy where an initially high DR3-restricted responsiveness to *M. leprae* seems present which however may become suppressed subsequent to the development of tissue damage and disease (see chapter 6).

Furthermore, in addition to the mentioned skin test studies with different mycobacteria in RA patients and healthy controls, experimental studies using T cell clones from RA synovia and well defined antigens such as the recently cloned and expressed *M. tuberculosis* specific genes (35) may identify the relevant epitopes on the bacillus and the target auto-antigens, whereas functional *in vitro* studies may elucidate which DR4 associated class II determinants are responsible.

Once the nature of this HLA-disease association has been fully recognized, rational RA prevention and therapy is expected to develop such as the modification of antigens in order to select for non-arthritogenic T cells, vaccination with T cells to induce idiotype specific suppression (36) and immunomodulation by means of class II epitope specific or responder T cell reactive monoclonal antibodies, as has been demonstrated for experimental allergic encephalomyelitis (37-38) and murine systemic lupus erythematosus (39-40).

Acknowledgements

The authors wish to express their gratitude to the patients. Without their frank cooperation this study would not have been possible. Furthermore, the authors would like to thank Dr. B. Gervasioni and dr. R. Ravioli who selected the majority of the patients, the medical doctors and assistants who contributed to this project, Diënne Elferink and Javier Gonzalez for their help in collecting blood samples, Ieke Schreuder, Henk Nieman and their colleagues for HLA typing, Peter de Lange for analyzing the data, dr. R.J.W. Rees for supplying Leprosin-A, prof. dr. J.J. van Rood for his support of the project and Ingrid Curiël for preparing the manuscript. This collaborative project was a direct result of the "Acciones Integrades" programme of the Spanish Ministry of Higher Education and the British Council who sponsered much of the work. This study was also supported in part by the Foundation for Medical Research (FUNGO; grant nr. 900-509-099), the Immunology of Leprosy (IMMLEP) component of the UNDP/WORLD Bank/WHO Special Programma for Research and Training in Tropical Diseases and by the Netherlands and British Leprosy Relief Association (NSL and LEPRA).

References

1. Kaufman, J.F., Auffray, C., Korman, A.J., Shackelford, D.A., Strominger, J. The class II molecules of the human and murine major histocompatibility complex. Cell 1984; 36: 1-13.
2. Benacerraf, B. Role of MHC gene products in immune regulation. Science 1981;212: 1229-1238.
3. De Vries, R.R.P., Van Eden, W., Ottenhoff, T.H.M. HLA class II immune response genes and products in leprosy. Prog. Allergy 1985; 36: 95-113.
4. Möller, G. HLA and disease susceptibility. Immunol. Rev. 1983; 70.
5. Van Eden, W., De Vries, R.R.P. HLA and leprosy: a re-evaluation. Lepr. Rev. 1984; 55: 89-104.
6. Qvigstad, E., Scott, H., Thorsby, E. HLA class II restriction of antigen specific T cell activation. Prog. Allergy 1985; 36: 73-94.
7. Kagnoff, M.F., Austin, R.K., Hubert, J.J., Bernardin, J.E., Kasarda, D.D. Possible role for a human adenovirus in the pathogenesis of celiac disease. J. Exp. Med. 1984; 160: 1544-1557.
8. De Vries, R.R.P., Serjeantson, S.W., Layrisse, Z. Leprosy. In: *Histocompatibility Testing 1984* (Eds. Albert, E.D. *et al*), Springer Verlag 1984; 362-367.
9. Van Eden, W., De Vries, R.R.P., Stanford, J.L., Rook, G.A.W. HLA-DR3 associated genetic control of response to multiple skin tests with new tuberculins. Clin. Exp. Immunol. 1983; 52: 287-292.
10. Bloom, B.R., Godal, T. Selective primary health care: strategies for control of disease in the developing world. V. Leprosy. Rev. Infect. Dis. 1983; 5: 765-780.
11. Ridley, D.S., Jopling, W.H. Classification of leprosy according to immunity. A five-group system. Int. J. Lepr. 1966; 34: 255-273.
12. Paul, R.C., Stanford, J.L., Carswell, J.W. Multiple skin-testing in leprosy. J. of Hygiëne 1975; 75: 57-68.
13. Shield, M.J., Stanford, J.L., Paul, R.C., Carswell, J.W. Multiple skin-testing of tuberculosis patients with a range of new tuberculins and a comparison with leprosy and *Mycobacterium ulcerans* infection. J. of Hygiëne 1977; 78: 331-338.
14. Van Leeuwen, A., Van Rood, J.J. Description of B-cell methods. In: *Histocompatibility Testing 1980*. (Ed. Terasaki, P.I.). Los Angeles, UCLA Press 1980; 278-279.
15. Schreuder, G.M.Th., Van Leeuwen, A., Termijtelen, A., Parlevliet, J., D'Amaro, J., Van Rood, J.J. Cell membrane polymorphisms coded for in the HLA-D/DR region. I. Relation between D and DR. Hum. Immunol. 1982; 4: 301-312.
16. Stanford, J.L. Immunologically important constituents of mycobacteria: antigens. In: *The Biology of the Mycobacteria* (Eds. Ratledge, C., Stanford, J) Academic Press, London 1983; vol. 2: 85-127.
17. Ottenhoff, T.H.M., Elferink, D.G., Klatser, P.R. and De Vries, R.R.P. Cloned suppressor T cells from a lepromatous leprosy patient suppress *Mycobacterium leprae* reactive helper T cells. Nature 1986; 322: 462-464.
18. Nye, P.M., Price, J.E., Revankar, C.R., Rook, G.A.W., Stanford, J.L. The demonstration of two types of suppressor mechanisms in leprosy patients and their contacts by quadruple skin testing with mycobacterial reagent mixtures. Lepr. Rev. 1983; 54: 9-18.
19. Nye, P.M., Stanford, J.L., Rook, G.A.W., Lawton, P., Macgreggor, M., Reily, C., Humber, D., Orege, P., Revankar, C.R., Terencio de las Aguas, J., Torres, P. Suppressor determinants of mycobacteria and their potential relevance to leprosy. Lepr. Rev. 1986; 57: 147-158.
20. Hahn, H., Kaufmann, S.H.E. The role of cell-mediated immunity in bacterial infections. Rev. Infect. Dis 1981; 3: 1221-1250.
21. Thorsby, E. The role of HLA in T cell activation. Hum. Immunol. 1984; 9: 1-7.
22. De Waal, L.P., De Hoop, J., Stukart, M.J., Gleichmann, H., Melvold, R., Melief, C.J.M. Nonresponsiveness to the male antigen H-Y in H-2 I-A-mutant B6. C-H-2^{bm12} is not caused by defective antigen presentation. J. Immunol. 1983; 130: 665-670.
23. Le Meur, M., Berlinger, P.G., Benoist, C., Mathis, D. Correcting an immune-response deficiency by creating Eα gene transgenic mice. Nature 1985; 316: 38-42.

24. Yamamura, K., Kikutani, H., Folsom, V., Clayton, L.K., Kimoto, M., Akira, S., Kashiwamura, S., Tonegawa, S., Kishimoto, T. Functional expression of a microinjected E_α^d f3 gene in C57BL/ 6 transgenic mice. Nature 1985; 316: 67-69.

25. Zamvil, S.S., Nelson, P.A., Mitchell, D.J., Knobler, R.L., Fritz, R.B., Steinman, L. Encephalitogenic T cell clones specific for myelin basic protein. An unusual bias in antigen recognition. J. Exp. Med. 1985; 162: 2107-2124.

26. Panayi, G.S., Wooley, P.H., Batchelor, J.R. Genetic basis of rheumatoid arthritis: HLA antigens, disease manifestations and toxic reactions to drugs. Brit. Med. J. 1978; ii: 1326-1328.

27. Holoshitz, J., Naparstek, Y., Ben-Nun, A., Cohen, I.R. Lines of T lymphocytes induce or vaccinate against autoimmune arthritis. Science 1983; 129: 56-58.

28. Holoshitz, J., Matitiau, A., Cohen, I.R. Arthritis induced in rats by cloned T lymphocytes responsive to mycobacteria but not to collagen type II. J. Clin. Invest. 1984; 73: 211-215.

29. Van Eden, W., Holoshitz, J., Nevo, Z., Frenkel, A., Klajman, A., Cohen, I.R. Arthritis induced by a T-lymphcoyte clone that responds to *Mycobacterium tuberculosis* and to cartilage proteoglycans. Proc. Natl. Acad. Sci. USA 1985; 82: 5117-5120.

30. Walker, P., Savill, C., Cambridge, G., Colaco, B., Shipley, M., Lydyard, P.M., Roitt, I.M. Analysis of synovial fluid cell lines from patients with rheumatoid arthritis. Abstract British Society for Immunology, Autumn Meeting 1985; p. 109.

31. Holoshitz, J., Klajman, A., Drucker,I, Lapidot, Z., Yaretzky, A., Frenkel, A., Van Eden, W., Cohen, I.R. T-lymphocytes of rheumatoid arthritis patients show augmented reactivity to a fraction of mycobacteria crossreactive with cartilage. Lancet 1986; ii: 305-309.

32. Janossy, G., Panayi, G., Duke, O., Bofill, M., Poulter, L.W., Goldstein, G. Rheumatoid arthritis: a disease of T-lymphocyte/macrophage immunoregulation. Lancet 1981; ii: 839-842.

33. Waxman, J., Lockshin, M.D., Schnapp, J.J., Doneson, I.N. Cellular immunity in rheumatic diseases. I. Rheumatoid arthritis. Arthritis Rheum. 1973; 16: 499-506.

34. Andrianakos, A.A., Sharp, J.T., Person, D.A., Lidsky, M.D., Duffy, J. Cell-mediated immunity in rheumatoid arthritis. Ann. Rheum. Dis. 1977; 36: 13-20.

35. Young, R.A., Bloom, B.R., Grosskinsky, C.M., Ivanyi, J., Thomas, D., Davis, R.W. Dissection of *Mycobacterium tuberculosis* antigens using recombinant DNA. Proc. Natl. Acad. Sci. USA 1985; 82: 2583-2587.

36. Cohen, I.R., Holoshitz, J., Van Eden, W., Frenkel, A. T-lymphocyte clones illuminate pathogenesis and affect therapy of experimental arthritis. Arthritis Rheum. 1985; 28: 841-845.

37. Steinman, L., Rosenbaum, J.T., Sriram, S., McDevitt, H.O. *In vivo* effects of antibodies to immuneresponse gene products: prevention of experimental allergic encephalitis. Proc. Natl. Acad. Sci. USA 1981; 78: 7111-7114.

38. Waldor, M.K., Sriram, S., Hardy, R., Herzenberg, L.A., Herzenberg, L.A., Lanier, L., Lim, M., Steinman, L. Reversal of experimental allergic encephalomyelitis with monoclonal antibody to a T-cell subset marker. Science 1985; 227: 415-417.

39. Adelman, N.E., Watling, D.L., McDevitt, H.O. Treatment of (NZBxNZW) F_1 disease with anti-I-A monoclonal antibodies. J. Exp. Med. 1983; 158: 1350-1355.

40. Wofsy, D., Seaman, W.E. Successful treatment of autoimmunity in NZB/NZW F_1 mice with monoclonal antibody to L3T4. J. Exp. Med. 1985; 161: 378-391.

CHAPTER 9

GENERAL DISCUSSION: *MYCOBACTERIUM LEPRAE* SPECIFIC ACTIVATION OF HELPER AND SUPPRESSOR T CELLS AND ITS REGULATION BY HLA CLASS II GENES AND PRODUCTS.*

1. Helper and suppressor epitopes defined on *Mycobacterium leprae* by cloned Th and Ts cells from leprosy patients.

Leprosy is a chronic infectious disease caused by *Mycobacterium leprae* which is estimated to afflict 10-15 million people mainly in developing countries (1). Leprosy has been designated as a "model immunological" disease since the striking variety in clinical symptoms which can develop upon infection in susceptible individuals correlates with the immune response of the host against the parasite (2). The leprosy spectrum ranges from "high resistant" or polar tuberculoid leprosy (TT), characterized by few self-limiting lesions and strong helper T cell (Th) mediated immunity against *M. leprae*, to "low resistant" or polar lepromatous leprosy (LL) with numerous progressive lesions and *M. leprae* specific T cell unresponsiveness, presumably as a consequence of *M. leprae* specific suppression (1). In between those two poles variable degrees of tuberculoid or lepromatous features can be found in borderline leprosy patients (1).

M. leprae reactive Th cells are supposed to be responsible for acquired protective immunity and delayed type hypersensitivity (DTH) reactivity against the bacillus in healthy contacts as well as in tuberculoid leprosy patients. Detectable Th cell reactivity against *M. leprae* antigens but not other mycobacteria is absent in LL patients (1). This *M. leprae* specific unresponsiveness is thought to be a consequence of *M. leprae* reactive Ts cells, although hard evidence for this supposition is still lacking. A number of studies has suggested the involvement of Ts cells, macrophages and suppressor factors from adherent cells, but the results obtained have sometimes been contradictory and not easy to interpret (reviewed in 3-5). The most suggestive evidence for Ts cells perhaps comes from the study of LL skin lesions. These lesions are characterized by a predominance of CD8+ cells over the few CD4+ T cells, large numbers of macrophages loaden with intact bacilli and poorly organized infiltrates, whereas the opposite situation is found in TT lesions (6). Although suggestive, it is clear that this observation provides only indirect evidence in favor of Ts cells in LL leprosy.

* Tom H.M. Ottenhoff and René R.P. de Vries. Submitted for publication in slightly revised form.

In order to obtain more direct evidence for such Ts cells we have recently cloned *M. leprae* reactive Th (CD3$^+$CD4$^+$) as well as Ts (CD3$^+$CD8$^+$) clones in order to characterize the antigenic determinants on *M. leprae* which activate such T cells. Nearly half of the Th cells studied recognized determinants exclusively expressed by *M. leprae*, or in a few cases by 1-3 other mycobacterial species (7-9). This high frequency of (nearly) *M. leprae* specific Th cells was unexpected since so far relatively few monoclonal antibodies raised against *M. leprae* were found to be *M. leprae* specific (10). Other Th clones recognized crossreactive or common antigens shared by most or all mycobacterial species (7-9). Recently, 5 *M. leprae* specific proteins have been described which were defined by *M. leprae* specific monoclonal antibodies (10). These specific antibodies recognize proteins with relative molecular masses of respectively 12, 18, 28, 36 and 65K. The genes for these proteins – at least those parts coding for the antibody defined epitopes – have been cloned and expressed in *Escherichia coli* (11). If these proteins would contain the relevant antigenic determinants for Th cells, responsible for DTH and protective immunity, this would imply a breakthrough for the development of *M. leprae* specific skin test preparations and a *M. leprae* vaccine since such proteins in principle would then be available in unlimited quantities. Thus far, the only productive way of growing *M. leprae* bacilli has been the infection of nine-banded armadillos, one of the few species besides man in which *M. leprae* can proliferate. However, the thus obtained numbers of bacilli will remain limited and probably will be outreached by demand for vaccinations on large scale.

We therefore tested purified preparations of respectively the 12, 18, 36 and 65K *M. leprae* specific proteins isolated from *M. leprae*. These protein preparations could stimulate both *M. leprae* specific and crossreactive Th clones, and thus carried (multiple) distinct *M. leprae* specific as well as crossreactive Th cell stimulatory determinants (8, unpublished observations). These results suggest that those proteins indeed may be relevant for Th cell mediated immunity. Ts clones were isolated from a BL patient whose peripheral Th cells as well as several Th clones did respond to *M. leprae*. These Ts clones specifically could suppress Th cell responses against *M. leprae* but not the unrelated herpes simplex virus antigen or mitogen (9). The Ts cells were devoid of cytotoxic or NK-like activity and were irradiation sensitive. When peripheral Th cells were stimulated simultaneously with *M. leprae* and herpes simplex virus antigens, responses presumably induced by the latter antigen could not be suppressed, ruling out non-specific factors or effects as responsible for the observed suppression such as e.g. IL-2 consumption or binding by Ts cells (unpublished observations).

Interestingly, these Ts cells could also suppress autologous Th responses against other mycobacteria than *M. leprae*. Thus, the Ts cells may recognize a crossreactive suppressor epitope on *M. leprae* and other mycobacteria. In subsequent experiments, it was shown that these same Ts clones also suppressed Th cell responses against the mentioned *M. leprae* specific 36K protein preparation. This implies that in addition to helper epitopes this protein also may contain at least one crossreactive suppressor epitope. The existence of helper as well as suppressor epitopes on the 36K protein would closely parallel the situation for other immunogenic protein antigens (e.g. 12-15). An alternative explanation for the observed suppression however is that these Ts cells recognize dominant idiotypic determinants or *M. leprae* reactive Th cells.

An interesting observation was that the crossreactive Ts clones not only were able to suppress crossreactive Th clones but also *M. leprae* specific Th cell clones from the same patient (9). Although one should be careful in generalizing these observations to polar LL patients, it may well be that such crossreactive Ts cells are important in maintaining the *M. leprae* specific unresponsiveness in LL leprosy. The question which immediately arises then is why these crossreactive Ts cells would not also suppress Th responses against other mycobacteria. As mentioned, LL patients remain good responders towards other mycobacteria. It is intriguing that evidence is accumulating that such patients do not respond to the common antigens expressed by these mycobacteria, which are shared with *M. leprae*, but rather to the species specific ones that by definition are not shared with the leprosy bacillus (16,17; G.A.W. Rook, submitted for publication). Thus, if the above findings with regard to crossreactive Ts cells indeed may be extrapolated to LL leprosy, these Ts cells will not be able to suppress Th cell responses against the species specific epitopes of other mycobacteria than *M. leprae* as apparent from these *in vivo* observations, but in contrast can suppress Th cell responses against the crossreactive or common mycobacterial antigens, shared between *M. leprae* and most other mycobacteria as well as the *M. leprae* specific antigens. Studies in mice have suggested that antigen specific Ts cells can only suppress the relevant target Th cells when the suppressor epitope is expressed by the same molecule or fragment as the helper epitope (e.g. 13-15). This so-called "antigen bridging" model may provide one explanation for our observations: upon priming with *M. leprae*, LL patients will develop crossreactive Ts cells that may recognize crossreactive suppressor epitopes situated on molecules that also carry *M. leprae* specific or crossreactive helper epitopes. Both of these molecules fit an antigen bridge since helper and suppressor epitope are present on the same molecule, and consequently can induce suppression. Note that the latter molecule is expressed also by other mycobacteria, explaining the suppression of crossreactive mycobacterial Th cells in LL leprosy. Since however Th responses against the species specific antigens of other mycobacteria are not affected, one has to assume – reasoning from this model – that these species specific helper epitopes either reside on other molecules than the crossreactive suppressor epitopes, or on the same ones but on a sufficient distance to allow the processing machinery of the antigen presenting cell to separate those two epitopes. In both of these cases no antigen bridging and thus no suppression would be present. As far as we are aware, it remains to be seen however if suppression would occur if an helper and a suppressor determinant to which the individual has been primed during different immunizations by different antigens (in our case: a crossreactive *M. leprae* suppressor epitope and a species specific non *M. leprae* helper epitope) would be present on one molecule. The grafting of suppressor epitopes on molecules containing a helper epitope that is not expressed by the antigen from which the suppressor epitope originates probably will answer this question (E. Sercarz, personal communication).

A second model which would explain the lack of suppression of the non *M. leprae* species specific Th cells in LL leprosy is what we prefer to call a "molecular identity" model. This model postulates that the original molecule carrying both the helper and the suppressor epitope that were involved in the initial induction of suppression has to be represented to the Th and Ts cells in order for suppression to occur. In contrast to the common helper epitopes of other mycobacteria than *M. leprae*, the species specific helper epitopes of such bacilli by definition can never be situated on the molecules that were originally involved in the induction of suppression against *M. leprae* epitopes. Thus, Th responses against such species specific epitopes in this way could evade Ts cells. At present we do not know whether the Ts cells described here recognize suppressor epitopes or idiotypes or perhaps even other structures. Be that as it may, an important practical implication of these findings could be that the activation of such Ts cells in one or another way may place constraints on the use of those *M. leprae* protein antigens for skin test- and vaccine-preparations. If suppressor epitopes will turn out to be responsible for activating Ts cells, the selection of helper epitopes could offer a relatively simple way out. If however anti-idiotypic suppression would be the mechanism of suppression, such an approach might not be helpful. In addition, very little is known about the nature of putative suppressor epitopes. An unanswered question for instance remains whether a given suppressor epitope always is a suppressor epitope, to which then the immune response may be or may not be focussed under the influence of e.g. Is genes, or alternatively that as a consequence of genetic or environmental differences a certain epitope can be seen as a helper epitope by one and as a suppressor epitope by another individual. Besides the mysteries surrounding putative suppressor epitopes, it is not yet clear which helper epitopes are relevant for protective immunity and which ones may be preferentially involved in the induction of immunopathology. As pointed out below, the use of additional immunological vaccine constituents such as monoclonal antibodies against Ir or Is gene products or T cell subsets may offer one way of modulating the immune response. Another way of immunomodulation may be the preventive or therapeutical vaccination with T cell lines or clones.

Although those questions may still be unanswered, substantial and encouraging progress has been made the last few years on *M. leprae* antigen characterization. The further dissection and definition of the relevant protective and/or *M. leprae* specific antigenic determinants by combined molecular and functional approaches will be achieved probably within years, thus rendering rational prevention, therapy and control of leprosy a real possibility.

2.HLA class II restriction determinants for *M. leprea* reactive T cells.

MHC class II molecules carry restriction determinants (RDs) which in association with antigen can activate Th cells. These RDs probably are the products of the MHC class II Ir/Is genes, as they are involved in the restriction and regulation of antigen specific Th cell activation. Each of the three groups of HLA class II products – namely DP, DQ and DR – expresses RDs (ref. in 18), but the exact molecules as well as the epitopes involved have remained poorly characterized. We recently have shown that the main RDs for *M. tuberculosis* reactive T cells are associated with DR and not with DP or DQ (18). In addition, a new RD was found that did not correlate with the allelic DR specificities but was associated with
LB-Q1, a cellularly defined allodeterminant which resides on a DR molecule that carries a supertypic DRw52 specificity (19). Similar observations with regard to preferential DR and not DP or DQ restriction were made with *M. leprae* reactive helper T cell clones from leprosy patients (20, chapter 5). Since DR molecules have a much higher expression than DP or DQ molecules (21,22), these observations suggest that quantitative differences in the expression of class II molecules correlate with their function in the immune response (23,24). Two out of 36 T cell clones defined novel RDs on DP and DQ molecules. Besides quantitative also qualitative differences between the class II products may contribute to their role in the immune response as has been suggested by other studies (23,24).

It has been demonstrated in mice that only minimal alterations in the structure of the polymorphic domains of class II molecules have important consequences for the induction of T cell mediated immune responses. For instance, the substitution of a single amino acid resulted in the loss of the expression of RDs for several cloned T cells (25). Such substitutions may even completely change the Ir status of an animal as in the case of B6.C-H-2^{bm12} mutant mice; these mice differ in only three amino acids within the first I Aβ domain from the original B6, H-2^b mice, and consequently have become nonresponders to the male H-Y antigen (26) and beef insulin (27).

An interesting observation in this respect was made with regard to *M. leprae* reactive T cell clones, restricted by RDs on the DR$\alpha\beta_1$ molecules (defined by inhibition studies; two types of DR molecules are expressed by the DR4 haplotypes namely $\alpha\beta_1$ and $\alpha\beta_3$. The $\alpha\beta_1$ molecules carry the DR4 and Dw specificities, the $\alpha\beta_3$ molecular express the supertypic DRw53 specificity) (see chapter 5) expressed by DR4Dw13 positive antigen presenting cells (APC). DR4 behaves like a supertypic specificity for the cellularly defined Dw4, Dw10, Dw13, Dw14 and Dw15 specificities. As summarized in table 1, six different T cell clones revealed 5 different patterns of *M. leprae* induced responsiveness when tested on a large panel of allogeneic DR4 positive APC. Two patterns correlated respectively with the DR4 and Dw13 allospecificities whereas the other three apparently correlated with different Dw13 related epitopes. The most likely explanation is that these 4 Dw13 related patterns represent 4 different polymorphic RDs on the DR4Dw13 $\alpha\beta_1$ molecule. DNA nucleotide sequencing has revealed that in the case of DR4 β_1 genes only very few nucleotides differ between the distinct DR4 related Dw β_1 genes. All corresponding amino acid differences appear to reside in the first polymorphic domain of the β_1 chains between residue 67 and 86 (table 1) (28,29). Interestingly, this part of the molecule is likely to be placed on the outher face of the $\alpha\beta_1$ molecule (30) and therefore may well be involved in the expression of RDs. Our results not only demonstrate that the *M. leprae* reactive T cell clones

table 1

Proliferative *M. leprae* reactive Th cell clones recognize distinct DR4 or Dw13 related restriction determinants (20).

Dw phenotype of DR4[+] antigen presenting cell	amino acid residues DRß1 chain	Different *M. leprae* reactive Th clones of one DR4[+] Dw13[+] patient:					
		1	2	3	4	5	6
	67 70 71 74 86						
Dw 4		+	-	-	-	-	-
4		+	-	-	-	-	-
4		+	-	-	-	-	-
4	leu gln lys ala gly	nt	-	-	-	-	-
4		nt	-	-	nt	nt	-
4		nt	-	-	-	-	-
4		nt	-	-	-	-	-
10	ile asp glu ala val	+	-	-	-	-	-
13		+	+	+	[+]	[+]	[+]
13		+	+	+	-	-	-
13		+	+	+	[+]	-	-
13	leu gln arg glu val	+	+	+	+	[+]	[+]
13		nt	+	+	+	+	[+]
13		nt	+	+	+	[+]	-
13		nt	+	+	+	-	-
14		[+]	-	-	-	-	-
14	leu gln arg ala val	nt	-	-	nt	-	nt
non 4		nt	-	-	nt	-	-
non 13							

Notes

. Residue differences with Dw13 are underlined.

. nt= not tested.

. DR4 negative antigen presenting cells did not induce proliferative responses.

. Responses could be blocked by anti DR but not DRw53, DP, DQ or class I specific monoclonal antibodies (20).

distinguish precisely one (Dw13 versus Dw14) till four (Dw13 versus Dw10) amino acid substitutions on the $\alpha\beta_1$ molecules, but in addition show that a difference of only one residue (namely Dw13 versus Dw14) can result in the expression of at least 4 distinct RDs. Thus, mechanisms other than primary amino acid differences seem to be responsible for this unexpected RD polymorphism. We interpret these data as evidence for the formation of multiple unique conformational epitopes or RDs on the $\alpha\beta_1$ molecule as a consequence of a single amino acid substitution (see figure 1). Evidence in favor of the conformational nature of RDs has been suggested by a number of studies in mice (31,32). A recent elegant approach has been the transfection of different halves of the gene coding for the polymorphic I-Aβ domain into antigen presenting cells. The results suggested that separated amino acid residues from both halves of the polymorphic I-Aβ domain can contribute simultaneously to the formation of RDs, thus suggesting a conformational structure of such RDs (33).

The analysis of the structure of HLA class II genes may be helpful in precisely defining possible disease and Ir/Is gene related differences in the sequences of patients compared to controls. One example may be a 15 kb DQβ DNA restriction fragment that is almost specific for patients with myasthenia gravis (34). This disease specific restriction fragment may code for an epitope on the DQβ chain which may be involved in the control of immune responsiveness to acetylcholine receptor antigens, for instance as a RD for Th cells (35). Another example is a 15kb DQβ DNA restriction fragment which correlates with an antibody defined DQ product (TA10) that is a marker for resistance to type 1 diabetes mellitus (36). Similarly it would be of great interest to know whether for instance the DR3 and DR4 associated DQ$_\beta$ sequences of TT and RA patients respectively differ from those of healthy controls, and how such differences actually would relate to immune regulatory differences. The transfection and site specific mutagenesis of such genes may resolve part of the mysteries surrounding the supposed disease related epitopes and RDs.

However, as evident from the unexpected complexity and polymorphism of the putative conformational RDs, the mere sequencing of genes may not provide the complete answer to the structure-function relationship of such RDs. The definition of such conformational functional epitopes by epitope specific monoclonal antibodies (see e.g. 32) would at first hand perhaps be the best strategy. If conformational RDs are specifically related to disease, it would then become feasible to selectively block the function of such RDs by the mentioned RD specific antibody, without interfering with other immune responses. Such a therapeutical application of course is also possible for "linear" RDs. The beneficial effects of *in vivo* treatment with MHC class II monomorphic antibodies have been established clearly in a number of experimental diseases (e.g. 37,38) but a major disadvantage of such monomorphic antibodies could be the blocking of all Th cell activation as an hazardous side effect.

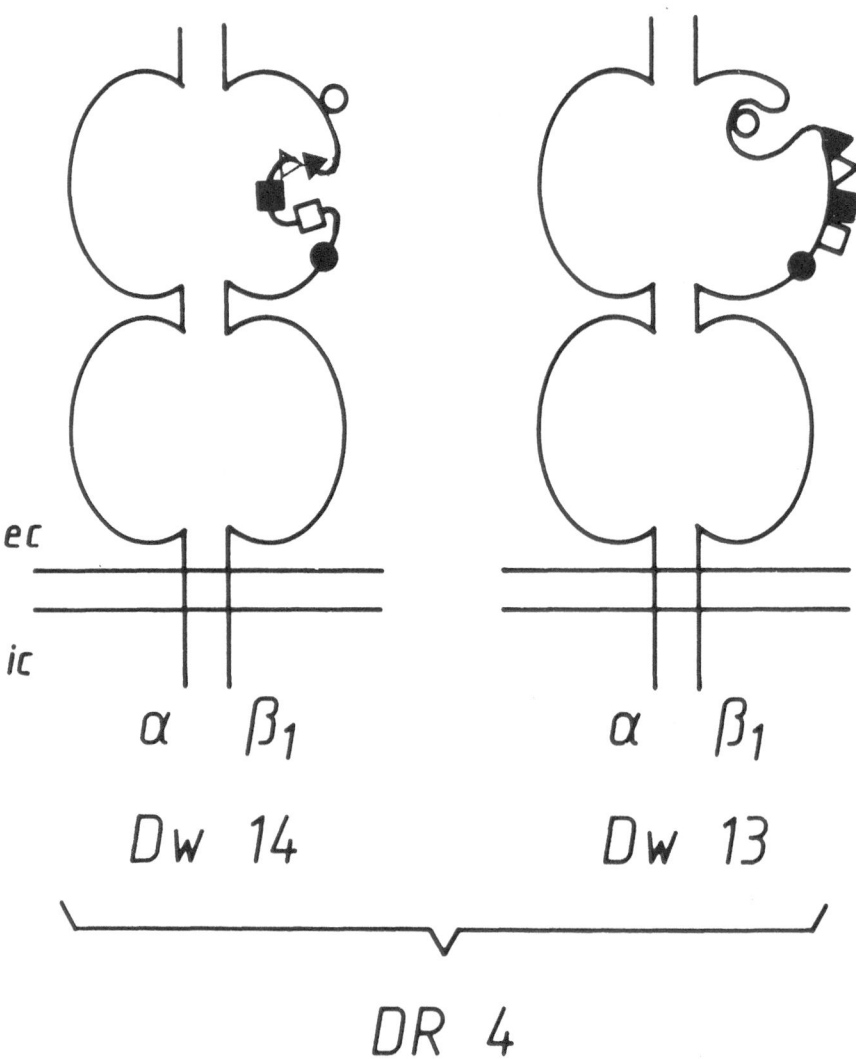

fig.1
Schematic representation of the possible conformational restriction determinants on DRαβ₁ molecu-les expressed by DR4Dw14 and DR4Dw13 haplotypes. Although Dw13 molecules differ in only one residue from Dw14 molecules (glu→ ala; pos. 74), Dw13 molecules express at least four Dw13 speci-fic restriction determinants for five *M. leprae* reactive Tₕ cell clones (see table 1), which are not pre-sent on Dw14 molecules.

- ala, glu : amino acid residue 74.
▲△■□ : Dw13 specific *M. leprae* restriction determinants
o : Dw14 specific *M. leprae* restriction determinant
ic/ec : intra/extra cellular

143

3.HLA class II Ir and Is genes and leprosy

3.1. Introduction

Immune responsiveness against specific antigens is controlled by a large number of polymorphic immune response (Ir) genes. In experimental animal studies, the majority of these Ir genes has been mapped to the major histocompatibility complex, the MHC (39). These MHC Ir genes control the response to so-called T cell dependent antigens by mechanism(s) that – although far from being resolved yet – may comprise the selection of antigenic determinants presented to T cells, the preselection of the available T cell repertoire or the differential activation of helper versus suppressor T cells (39). The products of these MHC Ir genes are the MHC class I and class II molecules (40). These molecules carry the RDs which in association with antigen have to be co-recognized by T cells in order for activation to occur (41). The extensive polymorphism of the MHC molecules and thus the RDs may lead to interindividual differences in antigen specific immune responsiveness, which on their turn may result in differential susceptibility to or expression of disease (42,43).

The observed associations between HLA class II alleles and several – mostly auto-immune – diseases are thought to reflect HLA class II Ir gene controlled antigen specific differences in immune responsiveness (44). However, despite the conspicuous resemblance to animal models, this latter assumption remains largely unresolved because the supposed triggering antigens essentially are unknown. Only few HLA class II linked Ir and Is (immune suppression) genes for defined known antigens have been described (45-47) but the relationship of HLA Ir and Is genes to disease has not yet been established, perhaps with the exception of the mentioned studies.

An important example of a disease in which HLA class II linked Ir and Is genes may be involved is leprosy. HLA class II alleles are associated with the type of leprosy as well as with the type of DTH reactivity against *M. leprae*, which both strongly correlate with Th cell mediated immune reactivity. This suggests that the mentioned class II alleles are markers for HLA linked class II Ir and Is genes (reviewed in 48-51) which thus most probably determine the type of T cell responsiveness against *M. leprae*. In order to study this HLA-disease model, we have isolated *M. leprae* reactive Th and Ts cells from TT and BL patients (see section 1), and determined which (and how) class II RDs are involved in the restriction (see section 2) and regulation (this section) of T(h) cell responsiveness against *M. leprae*. Here, we present a synopsis of this work and discuss its relevance for the understanding of the pathogenesis of leprosy and finally rheumatoid arthritis.

3.2. HLA-DR3 is associated with a regIr gene for M. leprae.

A number of *in vivo* and *in vitro* studies has revealed a differential role for HLA-DR3 associated genes and products in the immune response against *M. leprae* and related mycobacteria. The results of these studies are summarized and presented schematically in table 2. The association of HLA-DR3 with TT leprosy (compared to healthy controls) and of HLA-DR3 with high(er) respon-siveness both in patients and in healthy controls *in vivo* and *in vitro* suggests that HLA-DR3 associated high responsiveness to *M. leprae* and other myco-bacteria does not lead to TT leprosy in itself, but will do so only in susceptible infected individuals. This is consistent with previous results which indicated that HLA linked genes do not determine susceptibility to leprosy per se, but rather regulate the (tuberculoid or lepromatous) type of leprosy which develops upon infection in susceptible individuals (49-51).

Thus, DR3 is closely associated with an immune regulatory (regIr) gene for *M. leprae* that predisposes to tuberculoid but protects from lepromatous leprosy. In order to define more precisely the mechanisms by which this DR3 regIr gene may control Th cell responsiveness towards *M. leprae* in TT leprosy, we raised polyclonal Th cell lines against *M. leprae* (TCL_{lep}) and *M. tuberculosis* (TCL_{tub}) from DR3/non3 heterozygous TT patients as well as healthy controls. As shown in the same table, it appeared that the DR3 molecules were preferentially used as restriction elements by TCL_{lep} from healthy individuals as well as TCL_{tub} from both TT patients and healthy controls. This result seems consistent with the mentioned association of DR3 with TT leprosy and with high mycobacterial antigen responsiveness. Unexpectedly however, TCL_{lep} of TT patients displayed a DR3 associated low responsiveness. This low responsiveness was specific for *M. leprae*, DR3 and TT leprosy, thus suggesting an antigen specific disease related regIr gene effect. Preliminary evidence has been obtained in favor of DR3 specific *M. leprae* specific suppressor T cells which may explain in part this low responsiveness. The fact that TT leprosy has an essentially immunopathological appearance with the features of an excessive immune response such as granuloma formation, heavy infiltration of $CD4^+$ lymphocytes, peripheral nerve damage and destruction and relatively strong helper T cell reactivity against *M. leprae* (1) does not at all support the possibility that the DR3 associated low Th respon-siveness in itself accounts for the development of TT leprosy. In contrast, we think that this low responsiveness rather is secondary to the development of TT leprosy and tissue damage in an attempt of the immune system to suppress specifically and vigorously the initially strong DR3 restricted response that probably leads to auto-immune like tissue damage. TT patients will remain protected from developing lepromatous leprosy by T cell responses restricted via the other DR (non3) molecule since the observed (secondary) suppression probably is preferentially DR3 directed. Auto-immune reactivity in TT leprosy may – in analogy to experimentally induced auto-immune like diseases in animal models – be the consequence of inflammatory non-specific "bystander" damage

table 2

Association of HLA-DR3 with an immunoregulatory gene for responsiveness to *M. leprae* antigens.

individuals	DR phenotype	in vivo			in vitro			
		frequency in individuals.[57]	HLA haplotype inheritance[58]	skin test responsiveness to *M. leprae* antigens[59,60]	peripheral T cell response to *M. leprae* antigens[61]	Th cell* line raised to *M. tuberculosis*[61]	Th cell* line raised to *M. leprae*[61,62]	Ts cells to *M. leprae*[61]
tuberculoid leprosy patients	DR3	+++	+++	+(+)	+	+++	±	++?
	DRnon3	+	+	±	+	±	+++	+?
healthy controls	DR3	+	+	++	+(+)	+++	+++	?
	DRnon3	+	+	±	+	±	±	?

Notes

References from which the results are represented schematically are indicated. Studies were undertaken in patients and controls from a Surinam negroid population except for ref. 59 (borderline tuberculoid Ethiopian patients with a history of reversal reactions) and ref. 60 (healthy British individuals).

* The results shown represent the allelic preference for DR molecules to act as RDs for Th cells derived from DR3/DRnon3 heterozygous individuals. Thus, either the DR3 or the DRnon3 molecules served as the main RDs for these Th cells.

or alternatively true reactivity against auto-antigens, e.g. triggered by antigenic mimicry between *M. leprae* and host tissue components (52-56).

3.3. Is HLA-DQw1 associated with an Is gene for M. leprae?

HLA class II linked genes may predispose also to the development of LL leprosy (reviewed in 49-51). As summarized in table 3, several independent studies have suggested that HLA-DQw1 may be a marker for such a HLA class II Is gene for *M. leprae*. In contrast to the DR3-regIr gene for TT leprosy, no *in vitro* DQw1-Is gene effect for LL leprosy has been established so far: we could for instance not abolish nonresponsiveness against *M. leprae* in LL leprosy with DQ- and DQw1-specific monoclonal antibodies (unpublished observations). However, it is interesting to note that in another study, where DQw1 was associated with LL leprosy, helper T cell responsiveness could be restored by anti-DQ antibodies, strongly suggesting that the DQw1 molecules may be the products of an HLA-DQw1 associated Is gene (64). Our group has shown that DQw1 was associated with low peripheral T cell proliferative responses to PPD (65) (see table 3). Although the T cell donors did not originate from the population in which the associations of DQw1 with LL had been observed, these findings nevertheless may provide a clue for low- or non-responsiveness in LL, in particular since PPD and *M. leprae* share a number of antigenic determinants.

4. HLA-DR4: An Ir gene for *M. TUBERCULOSIS*-**specific antigens. A clue to the pathogenesis of rheumatoid arthritis?**

Rheumatoid arthritis (RA) is another disease, besides leprosy which we have discussed as a model disease, that is associated with a particular HLA class II allele, namely DR4 (44). Thus, DR4 may well be a marker for an HLA class II Ir gene predisposing to RA. The putative antigen(s) triggering the development of RA have remained largely unknown thus far. Recently, the results of skin test studies with different mycobacterial antigens have suggested that high responsiveness to *M. tuberculosis* but not to other closely related mycobacterial species is associated with HLA-DR4 (table 4). These observations thus suggest that DR4 is associated with Ir genes for RA and *M. tuberculosis* specific antigens. The intriguing possibility that one and the same Ir gene is responsible for both of these phenomena was suggested by the finding that in MHC susceptible rats *M. tuberculosis* specific T cells could induce a RA-like disease (66). Even more interesting is that this rodent model may indeed be extrapolated to RA since T cells isolated from affected joints of RA patients have been found to recognize *M. tuberculosis* antigens (67,68). Thus, RA may well be a disease closely related to TT leprosy (69). The understanding of the antigenic determinants, T cells

table 3

Association of HLA-DQw1 with an immune suppression gene for *M. leprae*?

individuals	DQ phenotype	in vivo			in vitro
		frequency in individuals.[63]	HLA haplotype inheritance[58]; chapter 2	skin test *non*-responders to *M. leprae* antigens[58, 59]	in vitro *low* T cell responses to PPD[63]
lepromatous leprosy patients	DQw1	+++	+++	+++	?
	DQnon1	+	+	+	?
healthy or non lepromatous controls	DQw1	+	+	+(+)	++
	DQnon1	+	+	+	+

148

table 4
HLA-DR4 is associated with an immune response gene for *M. tuberculosis* and rheumatoid arthritis.

DR phenotype	rheumatoid arthritis patients[44]	*M. tuberculosis* specific high skin test responders[17]
DR4	+++	+++
DRnon4	+	+

and mechanisms involved in the induction of and protection against these diseases has probably come nearby, and may offer rational prevention and therapy by means of modified antigens and T cells, and Ir gene or disease related T cell specific monoclonal antibodies, as has been demonstrated in experimental animal studies (e.g. 37,38,66,70).

Acknowledgements

The studies reviewed in this paper received financial support from the Dutch Foundation for Medical Research MEDIGON (grant nr. 900-509-099), the Immunology of Leprosy (IMMLEP) component of the UNDP/WORLD Bank/ WHO Special Programme for Research and Training in Tropical Diseases, the Netherlands Leprosy Relief Association (NSL) and the J.A. Cohen Institute for Radiopathology and Radiation Protection (IRS). We wish to thank Tiny van Westerop for preparing the manuscript.

References

1. Bloom, B.R. and Godal, T. (1983). Rev. Infect. Dis. 5: 765-780.
2. Harboe, M. and Closs, O. (1980). In: *Immunology 1980*. (Fougereau, M. and Dausset, J., eds.). Academic Press, London, pp. 1231-1243.
3. Rea, T.H. (1983) Clin. Exp. Immunol. 54: 298-304.
4. Nath, I. (1983) Lepr. Rev. (special issue): 31S-45S.
5. Bloom, B.R. and Mehra, V. (1984) Immunol. Rev. 80: 5-28.
6. Van Voorhis, W., Kaplan, G., Sarno, E.N., Horwitz, M.A., Steinman, R.M., Levis, W.R., Nogueira, N., Hair, L.S., Gattass, C.R., Arrick, B.A. and Cohn, Z.A. (1982) New. Engl. J. Med. 307: 1593-1597.
7. Haanen, J.B.A.G., Ottenhoff, T.H.M., Voordouw, A., Elferink, B.G., Klatser, P.R., Spits, H. and De Vries, R.R.P. (1986) Scand. J. Immunol. 23: 101-108.
8. Ottenhoff, T.H.M., Klatser, P.R., Ivanyi, J., Elferink, B.G., De Wit, M.Y.L. and De Vries, R.R.P. (1986) Nature 319: 66-68.
9. Ottenhoff, T.H.M., Elferink, B.G., Klatser, P.R. and De Vries, R.R.P. (1986) Nature 322: 462-464.
10. Engers, H.D., Abe, M., Bloom, B.R., Mehra, V., Britton, W., Buchanan, T.M., Khanolkar, S.K., Young, D.B., Closs, O., Gillis, T., Harboe, M., Ivanyi, J., Kolk, A.H.J. and Shepard, C.C. (1985) Infect. Immun. 48: 603-605.
11. Young, R.A., Mehra, V., Sweetser, D., Buchanan, T.M., Clark-Curtiss, J., Davis, R.W. and Bloom, B.R. (1985) Nature 316: 450-452.
12. Goodman, J.W. and Sercarz, E. (1983) Ann. Rev. Immunol. 1: 465-498.
13. Adorini, L., Harvey, M.A., Miller, A. & Sercarz, E.E. (1979). J. Exp. Med. 150: 293-306.
14. Oki, A. and Sercarz, E. (1985). J. Exp. Med. 161: 897-911.
15. Krzych, U., Fowler, A.V. and Sercarz, E. (1985) J. Exp. Med. 162: 311-323.
16. Smelt, A.H.M., Rees, R.J.W. and Liew, F.Y. (1981) Clin. Exp. Immunol. 44: 507-511.
17. Ottenhoff, T.H.M., Torres, P., Terencio de las Aguas, J., Fernandez, R., Van Eden, W., De Vries, R.R.P. and Stanford, J.L. (1986) Lancet ii: 310-313.
18. Ottenhoff, T.H.M., Elferink, D.G., Hermans, J. and De Vries, R.R.P. (1985). Human Immunol. 13: 105-116.
19. Ottenhoff, T.H.M., Elferink, D.G., Termijtelen, A., Koning F. and De Vries, R.R.P. (1985). Human Immunol. 13: 117-123.
20. Ottenhoff, T.H.M., Neuteboom, S., Elferink, D.G. and De Vries, R.R.P. J. Exp. Med., accepted for publication.
21. Sanchez-Perez, M. and Shaw, S. (1985). In: *Human class II - histocompatibility antigens*. (Ferrone, S. *et al*, eds.) Springer Verlag, New York, in press.
22. Koning, F., Giphart, M.J., Dobbe, L. and Bruning, H. Human Immunol. in press.
23. Janeway, C.A., Bottomly, K., Babich, J., Conrad, P., Conzen, S., Jones, B., Kaye, J., Katz, M., McVay, L., Murphy, D.B. and Tite, J. (1984). Immunol. Today 5: 99-105.
24. Bontrop, R.E., Ottenhoff, T.H.M., Van Miltenburg, R., Elferink, B.G., De Vries, R.R.P. and Giphart, M.J. (1985). Eur. J. Immunol. 16: 133-138.
25. Brown, M.A., Glimcher, L.A., Nielsen, E.A., Paul, W.E. and Germain, R.N. (1986) Science 231: 255-258.
26. De Waal, L.P., De Hoop, J., Stukart, M.J., Gleichmann, H., Melvold, R. and Melief, C.J.M. (1983). J. Immunol. 130: 665-670.
27. Lin, C., Rosenthal, A.S., Passmore, H.C. and Hansen, T.H. (1981). Proc. Natl. Acad. Sci. USA 78: 6406-6410.
28. Cairns, J.S., Curtsinger, J.M., Dahl, C.A., Freeman, S., Alter, B.J. and Bach, F.H. (1985). Nature 317: 166-168.
29. Gregersen, P.K., Shen, M., Song, Q-L., Merryman, P., Degar, S., Seki, T., Maccari, J., Goldberg, D., Murphy, H., Schwenzer, J., Wang, C.Y., Winchester, R.J., Nepom, G.T. and Silver, J. (1986). Proc. Natl. Acad. Sci. USA 83: 2642-2646.

150

30. Norcross, M.A. and Kanehisa, M. (1985). Scand. J. Immunol. 21: 511-523.
31. Kimoto, M. and Fathman, C.G. (1981). J. Exp. Med. 153: 375-385.
32. Lerner, E.A., Matis, L.A., Janeway, C.A., Jones, P.P., Schwartz, R.H. and Murphy, D.B. (1980). J. Exp. Med. 152: 1085-1101.
33. Lechler, R.I., Ronchese, F., Braunstein, N.S. and Germain, R.N. (1986). J. Exp. Med. 163: 678-696.
34. Bell, J., Rassenti, L., Smoot, S., Smith, K., Newby, C., Hohlfeld, R., Toyka, K., McDevitt, H.O. and Steinman, L. (1986). Lancet i: 1058-1060.
35. Hohlfeld, R., Conti-Tranconi, B., Kalies, I., Bertrams, J. and Toyka, K.V. (1985) J. Immunol. 135: 2393-2399.
36. Schreuder, G.M.Th., Tilanus, M.G.J., Bontrop, R.E., Bruining, G.J., Giphart, M.J., Van Rood, J.J. and De Vries, R.R.P. J. Exp. Med. in press.
37. Steinman, L., Rosenbaum, J.T., Sriram,S. and McDevitt, H.O. (1981) Proc. Natl. Acad. Sci. USA 78: 7111-7114.
38. Adelman, N.E., Watling, D.L. and McDevitt, H.O. (1983). J. Exp. Med. 158: 1350-1355.
39. Schwartz, R.H. (1986). Adv. Immunol. 38: 31-202.
40. Mengle-Gaw, L. and McDevitt, H.O. (1985) Ann. Rev. Immunol. 3: 367-396.
41. Schwartz, R.H. (1985). Ann. Rev. Immunol. 3: 237-262.
42. Zinkernagel, R.M., Pfau, C.J., Hengartner, H. and Althage, A. (1985). Nature 316: 814-817.
43. Kast, W.M., Bronkhorst, A.M., De Waal, L.P. and Melief, C.J.M. J. Exp. Med. in press.
44. Svejgaard, A., Platz, P. and Ryder, L.P. (1983). Immunol. Rev. 70: 193-218.
45. Sasazuki, T., Nishimura, Y., Muto, M. and Ohta, N. (1983). Immunol. Rev. 70: 51-76.
46. Sasazuki, T., Nishimura, Y. and Muto, M. (1984). In: *Immunogenetics. Its application to clinical medicine.* (Sasazuki, T. and Tada, T., eds.) Academic Press, Tokyo, pp. 21-37.
47. Scott , J., Hirschberg, H. and Thorsby, E. (1983). Scand. J. Immunol. 18: 163-167.
48. De Vries, R.R.P., Van Eden, W. and Van Rood, J.J. (1981). Lepr. Rev. 52 (suppl.): 109-119.
49. Van Eden, W., and De Vries, R.R.P. (1984). Lepr. Rev. 55: 89-104.
50. Serjeantson, S.W. (1983). Immunol. Rev. 70: 89-112.
51. De Vries, R.R.P., Van Eden, W. and Ottenhoff, T.H.M. (1985). Progr. Allergy 36: 95-113.
52. Van Eden, W., Holoshitz, J., Nevo, Z., Frenkel, A., Klajman, A. and Cohen, I.R. (1985). Proc. Natl. Acad. Sci. USA 82: 5117-5120.
53. Fujinami, R.S. and Oldstone, M.B.A. (1985). Science 230: 1043-1045.
54. Sun, D. and Wekerle, H. (1986). Nature 320: 70-72.
55. Crawford, C.L., Hardwicke, P.M.D., Evans, D.H.L. and Evans, E.M. (1977). Nature 265: 457-459.
56. Titus, R.G., Lima, G.C., Engers, H.D. and Louis, J.A. (1984). J. Immunol. 133: 1594-1600.
57. Van Eden, W., De Vries, R.R.P., D'Amaro, J., Schreuder, G.M.Th., Leiker, D.L. and Van Rood, J.J. (1982). Human Immunol. 4: 343-350.
58. Van Eden, W., Gonzalez, N.M., De Vries, R.R.P., Convit, J. and Van Rood, J.J. (1985). J. Infect. Dis. 151: 9-14.
59. Ottenhoff, T.H.M., Converse, P.J., Bjune, G. and De Vries, R.R.P. Submitted for publication.
60. Van Eden, W., De Vries, R.R.P., Stanford, J.L. and Rook, G.A.W. (1983). Clin. Exp. Immunol. 52: 287-292.
61. Ottenhoff, T.H.M., Elferink, B.G., Leiker, D.L., Lai A Fat, R.F.M., and De Vries, R.R.P. Submitted for publication.
62. Van Eden, W., Elferink, B.G., De Vries, R.R.P., Leiker, D.L. and Van -Rood, J.J. (1984). Clin. Exp. Immunol. 55: 140-148.
63. Ottenhoff, T.H.M., Gonzalez, N.M., De Vries, R.R.P., Convit, J. and Van Rood, J.J. (1984). Tissue Antigens 24: 25-29.
64. Kikuchi, I. and Sasazuki, T. (1986). Abstract 6th International Congress of Immunology, Toronto. p. 615.

65. Van Eden, W., Elferink, B.G., Hermans, J., De Vries, R.R.P. and Van Rood, J.J. (1984). Scand. J. Immunol. 20: 503-510.
66. Holoshitz, J., Naparstek, Y., Ben-Nun, A. and Cohen, I.R. (1983). Science 219: 56-58.
67. Walker, P., Savill, C., Cambridge, G., Colaco, B., Shipley, M., Lydyard, P.M. and Roitt, I.M. (1985). Abstract British Society for Immunology, Autumn Meeting 1985, p. 109.
68. Holoshitz, J., Klajman, A., Drucker, I., Lapidot, Z., Yaretzky, A., Frenkel, A., Van Eden, W. and Cohen, I.R. (1986).Lancet ii: 305-309.
69. Van Rood, J.J. (1984). Ann. Rheum. Dis. 43: 665-672.
70. Titus, R.G., Ceredig, R., Cerottini, J-C., and Louis, J.A. (1985). J. Immunol. 135: 2108-2114.

152

SHORT SUMMARY

After the general introduction into the immune system in chapter 1, chapter 2 gives a concise overview of the genes and products of the MHC, the role of MHC class II molecules in the restriction of Th cell activation and the genetic control of antigen specific immune responses by MHC Ir and Is genes. The evidence for human class II Ir and Is genes is discussed briefly. The reader then is introduced into the immunology of leprosy with particular emphasis on the immunogenetics of HLA class II genes and products in leprosy.

In the chapters 3 and 4, *M. leprae* specific and crossreactive antigenic determinants are defined by cloned Th and Ts cells derived from leprosy patients. Th cell defined *M. leprae* protein antigenic determinants will be relevant for the understanding of (i) protective immunity (rational design of a *M. leprae* vaccine), (ii) delayed type hypersensitivity (preparation of *M. leprae* specific skin test reagents) and maybe also (iii) immunopathology triggered by *M. leprae* antigens such as in tuberculoid leprosy. In chapter 4, the first cloned *M. leprae* reactive Ts cells derived from a (borderline) lepromatous patient are described. These Ts cells may be important for the definition of another category of *M. leprae* antigens, namely (iv) suppression inducing determinants and may be regulated by HLA class II Is genes (see chapter 2).

Chapter 5 addresses the functional definition of the restriction determinants on HLA class II molecules that are involved in the presentation of *M. leprae* antigens to Th cells. Antigen was presented to those T cells by large panels of extensively HLA class II characterized allogeneic antigen presenting cells. Inhibition of T cell responses was studied by using HLA class II specific monoclonal antibodies recognizing monomorphic or polymorphic determinants. The main restriction determinants for Th cells are shown to be carried by HLA-DR and not by DP or DQ molecules. It is assumed that quantitative differences in the expression of DR versus DP and DQ molecules are responsible for the observed preferential DR restriction. The data furthermore show that these Th clones may define several new restriction determinants and that those determinants may be expressed as unique conformational sites. The possible restriction determinants for Ts cells have yet to be identified.

Chapter 6 describes *in vitro* studies concentrating on HLA-DR3 molecules as the products of a *M. leprae* specific immune regulator (regIr) gene predisposing to tuberculoid leprosy. DR3 molecules carry restriction determinants which behave differently in the antigen specific activation of patient derived *M. leprae* T cell lines as compared to patient derived *M. tuberculosis* T cell lines as well as *M. leprae* and *M. tuberculosis* T cell lines from healthy individuals: a preferentially DRnon3 restricted T cell response against *M. leprae* is observed in patients in contrast to the preferentially DR3 restricted responses in the other three cases. Preliminary evidence suggests that suppressor cells may contribute to the observed *M. leprae-*, DR3- and patient-specific low T cell responsiveness.

A second HLA class II Ir gene that may be related to another disease than

153

eprosy could be identified when a group of Spanish Caucasoid leprosy patients was skin tested with several different mycobacterial antigens (chapter 7). HLA-DR4 was associated with high responsiveness against *M. tuberculosis* specific antigens. Since DR4 is also associated with rheumatoid arthritis and since a role for *M. tuberculosis* antigens has been suggested in the development of this disease, such an HLA-DR4 associated *M. tuberculosis* specific Ir gene may well be relevant for the pathogenesis of rheumatoid arthritis.

In summary, the results of the studies reported in this thesis show that *M. leprae* specific as well as crossreactive antigens are recognized by Th cells in conjunction with HLA class II restriction determinants. The latter reside predominantly on HLA-DR molecules. Ts clones from a lepromatous leprosy patient could be isolated for the first time. The results furthermore indicate that HLA-DR3 molecules are the products of an HLA class II regIr gene for *M. leprae.* This regIr gene predisposes to an important disease, namely tuberculoid leprosy, by regulating Th cell mediated immunereactivity against *M. leprae*. Another class II Ir gene associated with DR4 and specific for *M. tuberculosis* may well be relevant for the development of rheumatoid arthritis.